Epilepsy

100 Elementary Principles

Epilepsy

100 Elementary Principles

—— Third Edition ——

William H. Theodore MD

Chief, Clinical Epilepsy Section,
National Institute of Neurological Disorders and Stroke,
National Institutes of Health

and

Professor of Neurology,
Uniformed Services University of the Health Sciences,
Bethesda, Maryland

AND

Roger J. Porter MD

Vice President, Clinical Pharmacology,
Wyeth-Ayerst Research,
Radnor, Pennsylvania

and

Adjunct Professor of Neurology,
University of Pennsylvania,
Philadelphia, Pennsylvania

and

Adjunct Professor of Pharmacology,
Uniformed Services University of the Health Sciences,
Bethesda, Maryland

W.B. Saunders Company Ltd
London   Philadelphia   Toronto   Sydney   Tokyo

W. B. Saunders Company Ltd   24–28 Oval Road
London NW1 7DX

The Curtis Center
Independent Square West
Philadelphia, PA 19106–3399, USA

Harcourt Brace & Company
55 Horner Avenue
Toronto, Ontario M8Z 4X6, Canada

Harcourt Brace & Company, Australia
30–52 Smidmore Street
Marrickville, NSW 2204, Australia

Harcourt Brace & Company, Japan
Ichibancho Central Building, 22–1 Ichibancho
Chiyoda-ku, Tokyo 102, Japan

First published 1984
Second edition 1989
Third edition 1995

This book is printed on acid free paper

A catalogue record for this book is available from the British Library

ISBN 0–7020–1813–9

Typeset by Photo·graphics, Honiton, Devon
Printed in Great Britain by The University Press, Cambridge

To Judy and Candace

Contents

Foreword to the Second Edition

In the Foreword which I wrote to the first edition* of this book, I said that I found it to be a monograph with a difference which was in many ways quite fascinating. When Dr Porter originally approached me and explained his ideas relating to the book, I had to confess to having some reservations about the format which he proposed to use, but these were totally allayed by the content of the volume, which I warmly commended to a wide medical audience. Epilepsy is one of the commonest disorders of the nervous system with which all neurologists, as well as psychiatrists and other medical specialists, must frequently deal. Indeed all physicians in primary care, family doctors or general practitioners, however they are styled, as well as paediatricians, physicians in internal medicine and psychiatrists, need to have an understanding of certain fundamental principles relating to the diagnosis and management of this condition which so commonly confronts them in their everyday clinical practice.

Clearly this volume is not a textbook of epilepsy. Rather it is a comprehensive and detailed commentary upon 100 guiding principles that are of fundamental importance in the diagnosis and management of this common disorder. The presentation is detailed and explicit yet succinct and precise; the advice which the author gives is clearly expressed and he has plainly deployed in writing the book the fruits of his very considerable personal experience in this field.

This new edition includes a great deal of new information and many new and up-to-date references to the relevant literature. I know of no better source to which anyone interested in epilepsy, whether medically qualified or not, can turn to obtain cogent, wise and practical advice about the condition and its management. The author himself confesses that in the few years which have elapsed since the first edition appeared there have been important advances in the overall management of epilepsy, even though no important new anticonvulsant drugs have been introduced. There are a number of issues upon which he has changed his views in the light of experience and I believe that the practical examples which he quotes in case histories, describing his experience with individual patients, not only enliven the pages of the book but demonstrate to the full that this is a rapidly changing field in which both research and experience require changes in attitudes and procedures on the part of the doctor. The first edition was a great success and I am in no doubt that this much improved and updated version will be even more so.

SIR JOHN WALTON
Oxford

*Both Lord Walton and Dr J.K. Penry wrote Forewords to the Second Edition.

Foreword to the First Edition

The unique approach used in this volume on the diagnosis and treatment of epilepsy is deceiving. At first glance, the work may appear to be little more than a pocketbook of a hundred rules to be followed pedantically. It is much more than that, however. It is a basic source of well-referenced information about epilepsy for an audience ranging from medical students to experienced epileptologists. The former will appreciate its instructive approach and the latter will draw on the principles in formulating treatment plans for patients with epilepsy. These are essentially guidelines, not procedural dicta. Nevertheless, certain basic principles are crucial to the effective medical management of seizures. This volume offers a very personal but well-balanced interpretation of these principles. It also touches upon the no less important psychological concerns of epilepsy and explores the promising research advances that hold hope for improved care of persons with epilepsy.

Both students of epilepsy and clinicians working with epileptic patients have in this monograph a well-refined, practical treatise on the essential elements of the diagnosis and treatment of epilepsy. There is no better qualified author of this subject than Dr Porter.

J. KIFFIN PENRY
Winston-Salem, NC

Preface to the Third Edition

After two highly successful editions of this book as a solo effort by RJP, the addition of a second author seemed timely and appropriate. The infusion of new ideas and concepts was needed, especially in the areas of new drugs and surgical aspects of epilepsy. WHT has added this by writing new principles throughout the book, namely 8, 27, 28, 38, 43–83, 86–94, and 97–100. WHT independently wrote all the drug chapters to minimize the potential conflict of interest by RJP in his new role in the pharmaceutical industry.

Much has happened in clinical epilepsy research since 1989. To account for what is new, we have eliminated, consolidated, expanded, rewritten and rereferenced the book. The bibliography is completely updated.

We hope that this in-depth primer will be of use not only to neurologists and neurosurgeons, but also to primary care physicians, who will be increasingly called upon to diagnose and manage this difficult disorder. Should this book make a contribution to the care of patients with epilepsy, we will be most pleased.

W.H. THEODORE
R.J. PORTER

Disclaimer

The opinions and assertions contained herein are the private views of the authors and are not to be construed as official or necessarily reflecting the view of the National Institutes of Health, the United States Public Health Service, the Department of Health and Human Services, the Uniformed Services University of the Health Sciences, Wyeth–Ayerst Research, or the University of Pennsylvania. RJP is an employee of Wyeth–Ayerst, which markets lorazepam and primidone.

Acknowledgements to the Third Edition

We are grateful to our mentors in neurology, Drs Morris Bender, Robert Fishman and Melvin Yahr, and to our mentor in epilepsy, Dr J. Kiffin Penry. We also appreciate the energy and effectiveness of Ms Gill Robinson and her team at W.B. Saunders, UK.

Glossary of Abbreviations

ACTH	Adrenocorticotrophic hormone
AED	Antiepileptic drug
CBC	Complete blood count
CBF	Cerebral blood flow
CBZ	Carbamazepine
CBZ-E	Carbamazepine epoxide
CNS	Central nervous system
CPS	Complex partial seizures
CSF	Cerebrospinal fluid
CT	Computerized tomography
ECG	Electrocardiogram
EEG	Electroencephalogram
EMG	Electromyogram/electromyography
EMIT	Enzyme multiplied immunochemical assay
EPC	Epilepsia partialis continua
ETHO	Ethosuximide
FBM	Felbamate
FDG-PET	Fluorodeoxyglucose positron emission tomography
GABA	Gamma-aminobutyric acid
GI	Gastrointestinal
GTCS	Generalized tonic–clonic seizures
HDL	High density lipoprotein
HIV	Human immunodeficiency virus
IBE	International Bureau for Epilepsy
ILAE	International League Against Epilepsy
IV	Intravenous
LDL	Low density lipoprotein
LTG	Lamotrigine
MES	Maximal electroshock
MRI	Magnetic resonance imaging
MTS	Mesial temporal sclerosis
NIH	National Institutes of Health

PB	Phenobarbitol
PET	Positron emission tomography
PHT	Phenytoin
PTZ	Pentylenetetrazol (Metrazol)
SEEG	Stereoelectroencephalography
SEPS	Somatosensory evoked potentials
SPECT	Single photon emission computed tomography
SSPE	Subacute sclerosing panencephalitis
TRF	Thyrotropin releasing factor
TSH	Thyroid stimulating hormone
VPA	Valproic acid
WHO	World Health Organization

1 Approach to the Patient

1 The brain is just another body organ

Neurologists, neurosurgeons, and psychiatrists take pride in the domain that makes their specialties unique – the domain that makes man unique: the brain and its connections. Awesome and remarkable though it is, the human brain differs from other animal brains only in the degree of its complexity. Like other body organs, the brain is both vulnerable and resilient; it gets sick and then often recovers. Just as with other body organs, the symptoms of the brain's illness are unique to its function.

It is important for practitioners who deal primarily with the heart, lungs, kidneys, and other body organs to realize that neurologists, neurosurgeons, and psychiatrists do not have a monopoly on understanding the brain. Primary care physicians (family doctors) should be aware of the fundamentals of diagnosis and therapy in medical neurology. Just as some knowledge of psychiatry is a necessary everyday requisite in the practice of most physicians, a basic understanding of neurology is essential for effective patient care.

Epileptic seizures are but one of the many symptoms of a sick brain. The patient with epilepsy should be viewed as a person with a brain that malfunctions intermittently. The physician should approach the epileptic patient in the same way that he would approach a patient with transient cardiac arrhythmias, that is, with matter-of-fact attention to the diagnostically and therapeutically important details. Although patients with difficult and complicated problems may require the attention of a specialist, many patients with seizures can be treated by the primary care physician who has a firm grasp of the elementary principles of the diagnosis and management of epilepsy.

2 Assume that every patient with epilepsy wants to get well

Despite years of frustration, patients with difficult seizure problems are almost always hopeful of discovering something new – a new doctor, a new medication, a new procedure – that will enable them to lead a normal life. Although the physician must carefully temper optimism about any new therapy, most patients are willing to try a new regimen in the hope of achieving better seizure control. It is, therefore, incumbent on the physician to offer the best possible therapy. Improvements lost while trying a new regimen are usually (although not always) regained by returning to the former treatment program if the new regimen is a failure; thus the fear of trying something new should be allayed. Although the practitioner must be especially wary of the possibility of life-threatening generalized tonic–clonic status epilepticus when a new regimen is introduced, such an event is almost always avoidable if therapeutic plasma levels of phenytoin and/or carbamazepine are maintained and if changes are not made too rapidly.

Patients with severe seizures naturally become depressed when neither renewed hope nor new approaches are offered. There are indeed many patients who have uncontrolled seizures, but they deserve thorough evaluation in a referral center before their condition is considered refractory.

3 Concealing the diagnosis usually causes more harm than it avoids

In a small and fortunately diminishing number of patients, the family may be advised not to tell the patient, usually a child, the correct diagnosis, that is, seizures or epilepsy. Clearly, patients who have epilepsy must be considered individually, but most affected individuals are much better off if they are given an early explanation of both the nature of the disorder and the potential prejudices that they may encounter in society. If secrecy is attempted, the whole family must 'live a lie', with constant fear that the truth will suddenly emerge; this fear may shatter the patient psychologically. The resulting pressure on the family can be so severe that the patient suffers greater harm from the secret-keeping process than the truth would ever have caused.

Parents may be particularly likely to mislead their children about the diagnosis, perhaps because they fear prejudice and ridicule in school. However, it is much better to prepare a child, as well as teachers and other students, for the possibility that seizures may occur than to hope blindly that nothing will happen. The Epilepsy Foundation of America has developed several successful educational programs for presentation in schools with students who suffer from seizures.

Finally, the patient's ignorance of the truth can damage the relationship between the patient and his doctor (Riley, 1980).

---

4 Patients with refractory epilepsy require the resources of a comprehensive epilepsy center

---

Armed with the knowledge that many seizure problems are controllable and that most patients are willing to try new approaches, the physician should not hesitate to attack the problem with vigor. Just as with any other disorder, the physician needs: (1) to establish the diagnosis, (2) to set a therapeutic goal, (3) to define the best and safest plan to reach this goal, and (4) to proceed with the plan. If the patients are seen frequently and if appropriate changes are made slowly and deliberately, very few are likely to experience more than a slight increase in seizure frequency during medication changes.

Every patient with uncontrolled epilepsy, however, should have the satisfaction of knowing that all measures capable of producing improvement have been exhausted. Although most diagnostic and therapeutic possibilities can be adequately evaluated by the primary care physician or neurologist, specialized investigation and management can occasionally lead to revision of the diagnosis of epilepsy, a better pharmacologic regimen, or the use of surgical therapy; a dramatic improvement may be the result.

There are outstanding clinics and university centers in the United States to which appropriate referrals can be made. Patients and others interested in client information and referral services in the United States may wish to write to the Epilepsy Foundation of America, 4351 Garden City Drive, Landover, Maryland 20785 USA or utilize (in the US) the foundation's toll-free number, 1-800-EFA-1000. Physicians and other professionals who wish to utilize the foundation's National Epilepsy Library should call 1-800-EFA-4050. The main office is 1-301-459-3700.

Long-term comprehensive care is available in national centers in some countries (though not in the United States). Such centers provide not only long-term hospitalization for proper evaluation and treatment of epilepsy but also support eventual deinstitutionalization to the maximum extent possible. In addition to such centers, there are many outstanding clinics and hospitals throughout the world in which patients with refractory seizures can be definitively evaluated.

Information on the location of specialized epilepsy centers and clinics can be obtained from the national or local voluntary or professional epilepsy society. The national chapters of the International League Against Epilepsy and the International Bureau for Epilepsy are listed in the Appendix. If unable to locate the society in your region or country, up-to-date addresses of the local societies around the world are available from the Epilepsy Foundation of America (address above).

2 Diagnosis: Causes of Epilepsy

> ## 5 There are multiple levels of diagnosis in every patient with epileptic seizures; all are important

At a fundamental clinical level, the etiologic diagnosis involves identification of the cause of the epileptic seizures. At a more superficial yet therapeutically important level, the seizure diagnosis is based on the nature of the seizure type. These two diagnostic levels are often combined with other criteria (Table 5.1 and Figure 5.1) to provide the epilepsy syndrome diagnosis; an epileptic syndrome may be defined as a disorder characterized by a cluster of signs and symptoms customarily occurring together (Commission on Classification and Terminology of the International League Against Epilepsy, 1989). Classification concepts are further discussed in Principle 12.

The search for all three levels of diagnosis is necessary for the proper care of

Table 5.1 Data needed to provide a syndrome diagnosis

I. Information on *etiology*
    A. Etiologic diagnosis is either definitively known or definitively unobtainable (idiopathic), *or,*
    B. Etiologic diagnosis is suggested by some of the following:
        1. Neurological history, including age of onset and family history
        2. Neurologic examination
        3. Electroencephalogram
        4. Radiologic (and related) examinations
        5. Other tests, including psychological examinations

II. Information on *seizure type*
    A. Seizure type is definitively known, *or,*
    B. Seizure type is suggested by some of the following:
        1. Neurological history, including age of onset
        2. Neurological examination
        3. Direct or indirect (i.e., videotape) observation of a seizure
        4. Electroencephalogram, ictal and interictal
        5. Other tests, as above

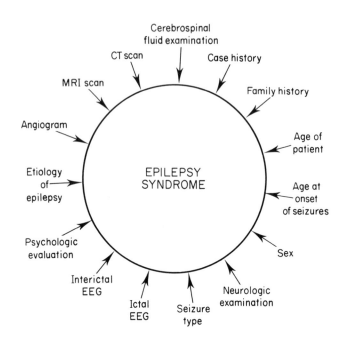

Figure 5.1 The epileptic syndrome diagnosis is achieved by evaluating all factors relevant to the patient. This view of the syndrome diagnosis is complementary to that of Table 5.1.

the patient with epilepsy. Failure to establish the etiologic diagnosis means that some patients will continue to have seizures because of undiagnosed brain lesions, e.g., a brain tumor. Failure to establish the seizure diagnosis means that some patients will continue to have seizures because the therapy is incorrect, e.g., absence seizures are mistaken for complex partial seizures and the incorrect medication is prescribed. Failure to establish the syndrome diagnosis will prevent the physician from understanding the prognosis and duration of therapy, e.g., mistaking juvenile myoclonic epilepsy (benign course) for progressive myoclonic epilepsy (malignant course). There is a clear relationship among the etiologic, seizure, and syndromic diagnoses; the first two are subsets of the last as noted in Table 5.1. Also, the etiologic diagnosis may contribute to the seizure diagnosis and vice versa. Although the etiologic diagnosis often cannot be established with certainty, the seizure diagnosis can almost always be determined. It is from the base of knowledge outlined in Table 5.1 that the physician establishes the syndromic diagnosis; in graphic form, this task is accomplished as described in Figure 5.1.

To understand better the relationship between the etiologic and the seizure diagnoses, one might consider a limited analogy to bacterial pneumonia in a setting of underlying lung cancer. The patient might have pneumococcal or staphylcoccal or *Pseudomonas* pneumonia, each requiring a different therapy.

Treating the pneumonia in this case is much like treating the different types of seizures with different antiepileptic drugs. The patient's fundamental (etiologic) diagnosis, however, is the cancer; the pneumonia is a complication or symptom of the fundamental etiologic problem, much as the seizure is symptomatic of an underlying etiology.

Clearly, it is just as inappropriate to say simply that a patient has seizures without giving a definitive seizure description as it is to say that a patient has pneumonia without naming the responsible organism. Equally important, of course, is the cause of the seizures, although the etiology unfortunately remains unknown in many patients with epilepsy. When possible, all of this information should be combined to provide an epilepsy syndrome diagnosis.

---

6 **The etiologic diagnosis, the seizure diagnosis, and the syndrome diagnosis can often be obtained from the patient's medical history**

As noted by Reiser (1978), the reverence of modern clinical medicine for objective evidence – data sensed and generated by machines and interpreted by technicians and specialists – has led to skepticism about the patient's subjective statements and distrust of subjective clinical judgments.

Although objective information plays an increasing role in diagnosis and therapy, the vast storehouse of data, however flawed, that is available directly from the patient must not be overlooked. The experienced physician need not listen to a rambling, disorganized monologue – quite the contrary. There are certain facts critical to the diagnosis of epilepsy that may only be revealed by interrogation. Although every doctor has an individual interviewing technique, some questions are indispensable. First, one must obtain a detailed description of the seizures. Many patients are not prepared for this line of questioning; others will give a terminology-oriented description, using such terms as 'petit mal' or 'temporal lobe'. The doctor must reorient the patient to more fundamental, descriptive terms (Porter, 1983). The doctor may begin by asking the patient 'What is the first thing that happens in a typical seizure?' Patients with simple partial seizures (or auras) will be able to describe the entire event by themselves in logical sequence. Patients with complex partial seizures will need assistance, either from persons who have seen the attacks or from a knowledge of what they have been told. The doctor may ask, for example, 'What do other people see when you have a seizure? What do they observe?' Finally, it is important to learn whether the attack ends abruptly or whether it tapers into a postictal state. One good question is 'Do you feel bad or tired after an attack?' A positive response strongly suggests the presence of an abnormal postictal state; such attacks are unlikely to be absence attacks, for example (Porter, 1983).

It is not usually necessary, except when psychogenic seizures are considered in the differential diagnosis, to obtain a detailed description of generalized tonic–clonic (grand mal) seizures; such seizures tend to be stereotyped, and are often secondary to a wide variety of more fundamental seizure types. Generalized tonic–clonic seizures are relatively easily controlled in most patients.

This history-taking process should, in most cases, lead to the seizure diagnosis (Chapter 3). The seizure diagnosis may greatly aid in establishing the etiologic diagnosis; determining the seizure type will even tell whether or not the etiology is likely to be uncovered at all. A ten-year-old girl with 35 attacks per day of sudden unresponsiveness, eyelid blinking, and lip smacking, lasting 10 to 15 seconds each, followed by instantaneous return to normal mental function, will almost certainly have absence seizures with clonic motion and automatisms (Principles 21 and 22); the etiologic diagnosis will likely remain obscure in this syndrome of childhood absence epilepsy. A forty-year-old man with daily parox-ysmal attacks of a bad odor followed by lip smacking and fumbling and then several minutes of postictal confusion and lethargy has complex partial seizures with a simple partial onset (Chapter 4); the etiologic investigation must consider tumor and other localized lesions in this syndrome of partial epilepsy. The medi-cal history often provides most of the clues to the correct diagnosis; it is, there-fore, invaluable and must receive special emphasis in the diagnosis of patients with seizures.

The medical history is easier to obtain if the patient is adequately prepared before the first visit to the physician and is accompanied on this visit by a relative or friend who has seen the attacks. When a seizure disorder is suspected, a letter can be sent to the patient before the first visit to the physician. This letter should instruct the patient to come prepared to:

1. Summarize the history of the seizures. Note when they first began, how frequently they occurred, and what types of seizures occurred.
2. Recall whether the nature of the seizures has changed since they first started. Be prepared to describe each type of seizure in detail. Ask people who have seen a seizure to describe it to you.
3. Try to remember the order in which medications were given, dosages changed, and new medicines started.
4. Recall which medicines affected the frequency of your seizures.
5. Recall the exact number of each type of seizure you have had in the past month.
6. If possible, have someone who has witnessed a seizure accompany you to the clinic.

If the patient comes with the above information, the physician is much more likely to understand the nature of the epilepsy.

PRINCIPLE 6

7   There are many etiologies of the epilepsies

Epilepsy can be caused by virtually any major category of serious disease or disorder of humans. It can result from congenital malformations, infections, tumors, vascular diseases, degenerative diseases, or injury. Although more than three-fourths of patients with epilepsy have their seizure onset before the age of 18 years (Commission for the Control of Epilepsy and Its Consequences, 1978), the incidence climbs rapidly again after the age of 50, reflecting disorders more typically seen in the older population (Hauser and Kurland, 1975). Any categorization of the causes of epilepsy should, therefore, attempt to distinguish between the causes in children and the causes in adults. Table 7.1 lists the major causes of seizures in children and adults. In addition, certain associations are worthy of note, i.e., both mental retardation and cerebral palsy provide a high relative risk of also having epilepsy, even though the etiology of the underlying disorder may not be known. If both mental retardation and cerebral palsy are present, the risk is even greater (Hauser and Hesdorffer, 1990).

In a substantial proportion of patients, the etiology of the seizures remains undetected. Future scientific advances are likely to identify two principal causes of epilepsy in this population. The first of these is inherited susceptibility. Although there has long been considerable evidence that absence seizures, for example, are an expression of an autosomal dominant gene (Metrakos and Metrakos, 1961), and although the role of genetic factors in epilepsy was, as recently as a decade ago, almost wholly unexplored (Newmark and Porter, 1982), new molecular genetic investigations have uncovered the chromosomal locations of seven epilepsy genes, with more likely to be identified in the near future (Delgado-Escueta, personal communication). One of the most impressive collaborations, for example, has been the combined population and molecular studies of Juvenile Myoclonic Epilepsy, the gene for which has been localized to the short arm of chromosome six (Delgado-Escueta *et al.*, 1984, 1989, 1994).

Table 7.1 Important causes of seizures in children and adults

Infants and children	Adults
No definite cause determined	No definite cause determined
Birth and neonatal injuries	Vascular lesions
Vascular insults (other than above)	Head trauma
Congenital or metabolic disorders	Drug or alcohol abuse
Head injuries	Neoplasia
Infection	Infection
Neoplasia	Heredity
Heredity	

From Porter (1980)

PRINCIPLE 7

Genetic investigations remain a priority investigative area, especially for patients with generalized epilepsies (Delgado-Escueta *et al.*, 1986). Future investigations will also begin to concentrate on the genetic aspects of partial seizures as well as the concept of 'genetic predisposition'. We need to learn why one patient has epilepsy after a head injury but another, equally injured patient, has no seizures. Head injury as an important cause of epilepsy is discussed in Principle 9.

The second possible cause of epilepsy in patients with seizures of unknown origin is chronic or subclinical infection. With the eventual identification of various agents that can cause disease without overt evidence of inflammation – such as Creutzfeldt–Jacob disease – and with the observation that many viruses, such as herpes, are present in latent form in humans, the following speculations are possible: (1) persistent infection must be considered in any chronic central nervous system (CNS) disease of unknown etiology; (2) the chronic infection may not have an acute phase or may not be accompanied by the systemic signs generally associated with acute encephalitis, such as malaise, fever, or even changes in the cerebrospinal fluid (CSF); and (3) it is likely that many causative agents of persistent infection have not yet been identified (Porter, 1980). In addition, the interaction between viruses and the human genome are just beginning to be understood. The concept of chronic encephalitis as a cause of epilepsy is not new, and derives from fundamental observations of Rasmussen *et al.* (1958); this syndrome has been termed 'Rasmussen's encephalitis', although the causes are probably very heterogeneous.

Finally, it should be noted that the effort to uncover the cause of epilepsy in a patient contributes directly to the etiologic diagnosis, but only indirectly to the seizure diagnosis. Classifications of either seizures or epileptic syndromes which are based on etiology alone have not proven useful (see Principle 12).

---

8 Ascertaining the etiologic diagnosis requires careful judgement in the use of special procedures

In the last decade, neurological diagnosis has been revolutionized by new procedures. Unfortunately, we physicians risk overwhelming both our patients and ourselves with technology. It is as important to know when a test will not be helpful as when it is necessary.

Evaluation of a patient with seizures can be divided into several stages. Each part of the evaluation should be designed to answer specific questions. In the first – the outpatient stage – the neurological examination, electroencephalogram (EEG), and magnetic resonance imaging (MRI) are performed; these studies provide most of the etiologic information. The second includes video-EEG monitoring, formal neuropsychological testing and psychiatric evaluation, while the third involves procedures designed specifically to localize foci for surgical intervention, including functional imaging tests (see Chapter 15).

Stage 1

Patients presenting with seizures may have almost any disease of the central nervous system, including some in which imaging studies are normal. It is very important to perform a complete neurological examination with an open mind. Detection of mild ataxia, for example, may suggest one of the myoclonus epilepsy syndromes. Moreover, epilepsy is a chronic disease. Even if no specific cause is found, the neurologist must have a clear picture of the patient's status at the outset of treatment. Before starting antiepileptic drug (AED) treatment, clinical testing of cognitive function and developmental assessment of children serves as a baseline for (1) detecting and following drug toxicity, (2) monitoring the adverse effects of the seizures themselves, and (3) following the progression of a degenerative disease.

All patients with seizures (or suspected of having seizures) should have EEG evaluations. Several tracings should be performed if initial records are unrevealing. Sleep deprivation may show epileptiform abnormalities not otherwise apparent, and inferior temporal (T1 and T2) electrode placements may be helpful when partial seizures are considered (Daly, 1990). Nasopharyngeal leads are now rarely used because of artifact contamination and discomfort.

Further tests will be suggested by the results of history, neurological examination and EEGs. In children, particularly those presenting with myoclonic or atonic seizures, evaluation for specific metabolic diseases may be appropriate, even though only a minority of patients will prove to have such a disease. Patients with primary generalized absence seizures do not need further evaluation at this stage. If focal epilepsy is suspected, an MRI scan should be obtained. Gadolinium enhancement is not necessary for initial screening (Cascino et al., 1989; Elster and Mirza, 1991). Focal gliosis and neuronal loss is the most common finding, but low grade astrocytomas, gangliogliomas, hamartomas, small arteriovenous malformations, and other lesions may be present (Theodore et al., 1990). The presence of mesial temporal sclerosis is not an indication for surgery if seizures are well-controlled. If a foreign tissue lesion is suspected, patient management will depend on its presumed nature.

Even if an initial scan is normal, patients should have repeat scans after an appropriate interval, since some slowly growing lesions may not be apparent on first seizure presentation. Moreover, imaging techniques are rapidly improving, with continuous increases in sensitivity.

PRINCIPLE 8

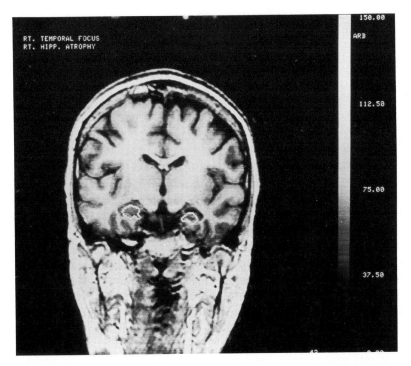

Figure 8.1 Right hippocampal atrophy in a patient with complex partial seizures and a right temporal focus. Hippocampal lobe outlines have been drawn for quantitative comparison of the two sides. The presence of atrophy usually correlates with mesial temporal sclerosis, although occasional patients may have both MTS and a tumor or other lesion.

Stage 2

In this stage the patient is referred to an epilepsy center. Patients in whom the diagnosis is uncertain, or do not respond to AED therapy, should be admitted for video-EEG monitoring to record their spells; this monitoring should be combined with frequent AED level measurement to ensure that therapeutic levels are present. At this stage the emphasis is on diagnosis; the seizure focus localization does not have to be verified. For patients with very frequent spells, outpatient video-EEG recording may sometimes be effective. Cardiac monitoring and sleep studies can be performed to exclude non-epileptic attacks (Chapter 7). Pseudo-seizures may be a diagnostic possibility in some cases (see Principle 33). Patients in whom the diagnosis is confirmed and are refractory to drug treatment can be considered for surgery; alternatively, the possibility of trying an experimental drug should be considered at this stage.

PRINCIPLE 8

Stage 3

This stage focuses on surgical evaluation. Additional seizures are usually recorded on video-EEG for localization of the seizure focus, if possible. In addition to the non-invasive tests performed in Stage 2, additional imaging studies including more detailed MRI, positron emission tomography (PET) and single photon emission computed tomography (SPECT), may be obtained (see Principle 90). PET and SPECT have no clinical role if surgery is not being considered. Neuropsychologic and psychiatric evaluation should be obtained. Arteriography, and the Wada test, or intracarotid sodium amytal test for language lateralization, as well as invasive electrode recordings, if needed, are carried out.

The following case shows the importance of periodic reevaluation and the impact of improved imaging techniques.

A 35-year-old librarian had had complex partial seizures for 15 years. Several CT scans had shown only left temporal volume loss. PET showed left temporal hypometabolism. Because the patient was right-handed surgical evaluation was not pursued and a series of experimental drugs was tried without improvement in seizure frequency; indeed, the patient had evidence of progressive neuropsychological impairment. An MRI scan then showed increased left temporal signal intensity and surgical resection was performed with intraoperative functional mapping; a disembryoplastic epilethelioma was removed. The patient has been seizure-free for three years, and has obtained a promotion at work.

---

9 Head trauma is the most common preventable cause of epilepsy

---

Most persons feel that epilepsy is something bad that happens to someone else. In the case of post-traumatic epilepsy, all are at risk. The risk is not trivial, and the impact can be devastating. Most civilian head injuries come from automobile accidents and are exaggerated by failure to utilize safety features such as seat belts which may limit the severity of the injury. According to Lewis et al. (1993), the factors (in children, at least) which predict post-traumatic epilepsy are (1) loss of consciousness, (2) low Glasgow Coma score, and (3) an abnormal computerized tomography (CT) scan. A disproportionate number of accidents and head injuries occur in the younger age groups, where life expectancy is long and the need for rehabilitation is greatest.

Annegers et al. (1980) ascertained the prevalence of severe head injury among a cohort of 2747 head-injured patients in Olmstead County, Minnesota, and found that 195 (7%) of these patients had suffered one or more of: (1) documented brain contusion, (2) intracranial hematoma, or (3) 24 hours or more of either unconsciousness or post-traumatic amnesia. After five years of follow-up, 11.5% of these patients had experienced 'late seizures', i.e., post-traumatic epilepsy. If one considers that, in the US in 1974 (from which the best figures are available), at least 400,000 head injuries occur annually (Kalsbeek *et al.*, 1980), and assuming that the proportion of severe head injuries is the same as in the Minnesota study, i.e., 7%, and assuming that 11.5% of these patients will have post-traumatic epilepsy, then more than 3,000 cases of epilepsy are added every year to the US population because of head injury. This figure is not corrected for the increase in population in the US in the past 20 years; also, if calculations for 'moderate' head injury are added to the above, the annual incidence of post-traumatic epilepsy rises to over 5,000 cases per year. Moderate head injuries are much less likely to cause epilepsy, but are very much more common than severe injuries (Annegers *et al.*, 1980).

Patients with post-traumatic epilepsy usually have localized damage to their brain; the chronic seizures are therefore usually partial, with or without secondary generalization. The attacks can be very difficult to control. In addition to epilepsy, personality changes and memory dysfunction often accompany severe head injury. The role of genetic predisposition in the development of post-traumatic seizures has recently been challenged (Schaumann *et al.*, 1994).

---

10 **Sudden, unexplained death remains a serious problem in patients with severe epilepsy**

'The danger to life in epilepsy is not great. Alarming as is the aspect of a severe epileptic fit – imminent as the danger to life appears when the patient is lying senseless, with livid, swollen and distorted features, and convulsions which almost asphyxiate him or her, looking "as if strangled by the bow of an invisible executioner", it is extremely rare for a patient to die during a fit. The chief danger of death in an attack is the liability to accidental asphyxia, in consequence of the occurrence of an attack during a meal, when food may get into the air-passages, or of vomiting after an attack with the same result, or in consequence of the patient, in bed, after an attack, turning on the face and being suffocated in the postepileptic insensibility.' Thus did Gowers (1885) observe that epileptic seizures are rarely associated with death but that some patients do in fact die, perhaps from various causes of asphyxiation.

Some studies confirm the overall increased incidence of mortality in patients with epilepsy (Hauser *et al.*, 1980), but since Gowers' time little new knowledge has emerged about the causes of sudden death in patients with epilepsy. Many reports have focused on asphyxia, perhaps because convulsions inherently cause respiratory embarrassment. A case report exemplifies the problem:

A 17-year-old girl was well until the previous year, when she had the sudden onset of viral encephalitis associated with multiple generalized tonic–clonic seizures, confusion, and lethargy for approximately two weeks. She was left with a residuum of memory loss and frequent generalized tonic–clonic seizures. A regimen of phenytoin and carbamazepine was gradually prescribed to maximally tolerated doses, and the patient slowly improved. She had returned to special classes in school, and her seizure frequency had decreased from an average of three seizures a week to one or two a month. She was found dead at home by her parents, her face buried in the pillow. An autopsy was consistent with, but not diagnostic of, asphyxiation.

Many have blamed pillows for suffocation of patients with nocturnal seizures, but proof is difficult to obtain. Those who speculate about this means of suffocation argue that the usual reflexes are not available to ensure an adequate airway after a generalized tonic–clonic seizure. In the postictal state, should the patient, already acidotic from the seizure, have his/her head buried in a pillow, the usual corrective tachypnea would be impossible, the acidosis would worsen, and fatal cardiac arrhythmia would result. Neurogenic pulmonary edema also has been implicated as a likely cause of sudden, unexplained death in epilepsy (Terrence et al., 1981). It has also been speculated that increased circulating catecholamines cause fatal cardiac arrhythmias in epileptic patients. Although a study of 338 consecutive patients with epilepsy did not reveal a predisposition to serious cardiac arrhythmias (Keilson et al., 1987), the smaller study by Earnest ei al. (1992) implicated arrhythmia as a primary suspect. As noted by Hauser and Hessdorffer (1990), the lack of a comparison group in most studies makes impossible any reasonable conclusion regarding the mechanisms of death in these circumstances.

Another, better documented cause of death in epilepsy is drowning. Although patients with epilepsy should be encouraged to enjoy a normal life, swimming must continue to be a regulated activity. Patients with epilepsy, especially those who have alteration of consciousness, should use extreme caution when swimming or boating; poor judgment can result in tragedy. Two simple rules can greatly decrease the likelihood of drowning: (1) never swim, boat, or play near water without a companion who can swim, and (2) wear a life jacket whenever it is possible and reasonable. If a seizure does occur in the water, the patient should be removed from the water and placed on his side, vital signs should be checked, and artificial respiration provided as necessary. Those who seem to have recovered should still be evaluated by a physician.

---

11 Neonatal seizures are a separate empirical group

Volpe (1981) stressed the need for better definition of the various clinical manifestations of seizures in newborns and recognized the importance of future clinical research in delineation of the precise relationships of seizure type to gestational age, etiology, response to therapy, and outcome. Neonatal epileptic seizures differ greatly from seizures in older children or adults. Convulsions are often encountered during the first few weeks of life and are often the presenting manifestation of serious neurologic dysfunction in the newborn (Rose and Lombroso, 1970; Lombroso and Holmes, 1993). For these reasons, neonatal seizures must be considered as a special diagnostic, therapeutic, and prognostic entity.

Only the most rudimentary aspects of neonatal seizures can be addressed in this volume. The earliest meaningful classification of neonatal seizures is that of Volpe (1981), who divided the attacks into five fundamental subgroups: (1) subtle, (2) generalized tonic, (3) multifocal clonic, (4) focal clonic, and (5) myoclonic. Although this classification has proven to be highly functional, a number of investigators have questioned whether many of the clinical phenomena observed in neonates – which have been attributed to seizures – are in fact epileptic. Mizrahi and Kellaway (1987) evaluated 415 clinical seizures in 349 neonates and constructed a somewhat different classification (Table 11.1), with emphasis on those attacks which had a 'consistent electrical signature'. Others suggest that unaided visual inspection of neonates may greatly underestimate actual seizure frequency (Clancy *et al.*, 1988).

According to Volpe (1981), subtle seizures are frequently overlooked; they consist of horizontal eye movements and eyelid blinking, oral automatisms, 'ped-

---

Table 11.1 Neonatal seizure types

I.   Seizures with a consistent electrical signature
         1. Focal clonic seizures
         2. Myoclonic seizures
         3. Focal tonic seizures
         4. Apnea

II.   Seizures with inconsistent EEG signature
         1. Motor automatisms
         2. Generalized tonic seizures
         3. Myoclonic seizures

III.   Infantile spasms

IV.   EEG seizures without clinical seizures

From Mizrahi and Kellaway (1987), with permission.

PRINCIPLE 11

aling' and similar stereotyped movements, and apneic episodes. Tonic seizures resemble either decorticate or decerebrate posturing, but are associated with diagnostically definitive eye signs, apnea, or clonic jerks. Multifocal clonic seizures are migratory clonic jerks without a 'march', and are seen especially in full-term infants. Focal clonic seizures are unusual, and do not always indicate localized injury. Myoclonic seizures are also rare, as are bilateral massive myoclonic jerks; some patients later develop typical infantile spasms.

According to Mizrahi and Kellaway (1987), focal clonic seizures are rhythmic twitchings with a time-locked central EEG sharp wave; they may be unifocal, multifocal, hemiconvulsive, or axial. Myoclonic seizures are 'single jerks or slow serial jerking', and may be generalized or focal. Focal tonic seizures are sustained asymmetric posturing of limbs or trunk. Apnea was described in one patient. Other events had no consistent relationship to EEG abnormalities.

Niedermeyer (1993a) combined several of previous classifications and created a hybrid classification which is very approachable (Table 11.2). He emphasized that neonatal seizures are often obvious and unmistakable but also may be subtle, hidden, or even debatable.

In the 137 patients studied by Rose and Lombroso (1970), hypocalcemia was the most common etiologic factor in such seizures (20%), followed by

Table 11.2 Common neonatal seizure patterns

Clonic	Focal (implying focal brain lesions)
	Multifocal (fragmentary, anarchic; must be differentiated from jitteriness)
	Hemiconvulsive (rare in newborns; more frequent in young infants – may be hemiclonic or hemitonic)
Subtle	Abnormal eye movements; mild posturing; oral lingual movements; pedaling and rowing movements; brief tremors, apneas (difficult to diagnose without EEG)
Tonic	Focal or generalized (resemble decerebrate posturing; often with abnormal eye movements, apnea, cyanosis)
Myoclonic	Often fragments of infantile spasms seen later in infancy (must be differentiated from Moro and startles of non-REM sleep)
Ictal apnea	May be combined with cyanosis and hypotonia
Absence-like	Staring with pallor and muscular hypotonia
Oculomotor	Upward eye movement ('eyes rolling up')
Further ictal manifestations	Slight finger contractions; alternating 'warding off' arm movements; sudden awakening with crying; eye opening; paroxysmal blinking; nystagmus; vasomotor changes; chewing; limb movements resembling 'swimming, rowing and pedaling'; abrupt changes in respiration, skin color, salivation

From Niedermeyer (1993a), with permission from the copyright holder, Williams & Wilkins.

PRINCIPLE 11

intracranial birth injury (15%); lesser, but still important, causes were central nervous system (CNS) infection, congenital cerebral malformation, perinatal anoxia, postmaturity, hypoglycemia. Volpe (1981), a decade later, noted that 60% of his cases were caused by perinatal asphyxia and 15% were related to intracranial hemorrhage; these findings probably reflect improvements in neonatal metabolic monitoring and control, although Volpe emphasized the presence of concomitant disorders in patients with hypocalcemia and hypoglycemia.

The approach to the newborn with seizures has become controversial. Some have suggested that treatment is urgent, especially if the seizures are continuous; emphasis has been on seeking the etiology and 'controlling' the seizures without delay, on the assumption – still possibly correct – that the seizures themselves may damage the child's brain. Other investigators, however, have inserted a note of caution, emphasizing that not all events that have been treated in the past are necessarily epileptic, and that treatment can only be justified for those events in which evidence exists for an epileptic cause (Mizrahi and Kellaway, 1987). A scoring system to predict neurological sequelae has been developed and evaluated (Ellison et al., 1986).

Should treatment be instituted, rapid loading with phenytoin or phenobarbital will usually suffice, although diazepam or paraldehyde may be needed in patients with status epilepticus (Fenichel, 1985). Loading doses of 15 to 20 mg/kg of phenytoin or phenobarbital are needed to achieve therapeutic levels in the newborn; furthermore, orally administered phenytoin is not predictably absorbed (Painter et al., 1981). Lorazepam may also be useful (Maytal et al., 1991).

The prognosis of neonatal seizures, as with many of the epilepsies, is greatly dependent on the underlying etiology.

3 Diagnosis: Seizures and Epilepsy

---

12 The classification of epileptic syndromes is different from the classification of epileptic seizures

---

There is a fundamental difference between seizures and epilepsy. A seizure is a finite event; it has a beginning and an end. Hughlings Jackson, in 1870, stated that a seizure is a 'symptom. . .an occasional, an excessive and a disorderly discharge of nerve tissue. . .' (Taylor, 1931). Epilepsy, on the other hand, is a chronic disorder. The World Health Organization (WHO) has stated that epilepsy is 'a chronic brain disorder of various etiologies characterized by recurrent seizures due to excessive discharge of cerebral neurons. . .' (Gastaut, 1973). Epilepsy is more a group a syndromes than a disease; 'the epilepsies' or 'epileptic syndromes' have arisen to classify *patients* and to emphasize the heterogeneity of these symptom complexes. The classification of epileptic syndromes is now becoming very useful to the practitioner even though it has proved much more difficult to devise than the classification of epileptic seizures. This principle will elaborate on epileptic syndromes (the epilepsies).

The classification of the epilepsies depends on our ability to determine a framework of similarity in patient characteristics – including seizures and many other factors. The earliest and most persistent subdivisions distinguish the epilepsies by dividing them into three groups: (1) epilepsy with a recognizable cause (symptomatic), (2) epilepsy with a suspected – but hidden – cause (cryptogenic) and (3) epilepsy without a recognizable cause other than heredity (idiopathic). The cryptogenic and idiopathic groups of patients have been gradually getting smaller with improvements in clinical diagnostic techniques and genetic investigations. The terms 'primary epilepsy' (meaning that the etiology is unknown) and 'secondary epilepsy' (meaning that the etiology is clinically identifiable) have also been used in a similar way to differentiate the epilepsies even though these terms present special semantic difficulties. Secondary epilepsy is a quite different concept from secondary generalization of seizures, with which it may be confused (Principle 20).

Following early efforts by Merlis (1970, 1972), the classification of the epilepsies was not vigorously pursued until the 1980s. In 1985, the International League Against Epilepsy published a new proposal for such classification; a revision was published in 1989. The fundamental observations are similar to those of Merlis and reflect the earlier success of the classification of epileptic seizures by beginning first with the partial/generalized concept followed by the etiology concept:

    I. Partial (localization-related) epilepsies
       A. Idiopathic
       B. Symptomatic
       C. Cryptogenic
   II. Generalized epilepsies
       A. Idiopathic
       B. Cryptogenic or symptomatic
       C. Symptomatic
  III. Epilepsies undetermined whether partial or generalized
  IV. Special syndromes

The next subdivision below partial/generalized and idiopathic/cryptogenic/symptomatic, especially for the generalized epilepsies, is the relationship of age to onset, one of the most important variables underlying the classification. Where appropriate, the classification progresses from the youngest affected group to the oldest. Relationship to age is most important in the generalized idiopathic epilepsies and least important in the partial symptomatic epilepsies.

Whenever possible, it is desirable to categorize a patient into an epileptic syndrome; a syndrome classification affords prognostic information for the patient that neither the seizure diagnosis nor the etiologic diagnosis can provide. The relationships among seizure type, etiology, and epileptic syndrome have been discussed in Principle 6. The classification of the epilepsies is, however, still evolving. The following is a summary, based on the above outline, of the most important and relevant syndromes as viewed by this author. The data come primarily from the 1989 Commission report.

Partial epilepsies, idiopathic

1. *Benign childhood epilepsy with centrotemporal spikes.* This syndrome typically occurs between the ages of 3 and 13, and is characterized by brief, simple partial hemifacial motor seizures; these attacks tend to secondarily generalize. A genetic predisposition is frequent and males are predominant (Principle 16).
2. *Childhood epilepsy with occipital paroxysms.* This syndrome is similar to the one above. Visual symptoms may occur at the onset, and some patients have an associated migraine headache.

Partial epilepsies, symptomatic

This group of syndromes, in which the etiology of the seizures is known or suspected, is largely characterized by the seizure type, which is very much determined by the locus of onset of the attacks. Two rare conditions, *chronic progressive epilepsia partialis continua of childhood (Kojewnikow's syndrome)*, and *syndromes characterized by specific modes of precipitation*, will not be further described here.

Included in this group, however, are syndromes characterized by simple and complex partial seizures as well as secondarily generalized seizures. Obviously this group encompasses the most frequent and severe epilepsy problems of adults. The anatomically designated syndromes are as follows:

1. Temporal lobe epilepsies.
2. Frontal lobe epilepsies.
3. Parietal lobe epilepsies.
4. Occipital lobe epilepsies.

Some of these epilepsies have their onset from multiple lobes, and some from unknown loci. These syndromes are still evolving. Although the medical therapy for all of these syndromes is usually similar, their individual recognition is important when considering surgical therapy for the patient's epilepsy (Chapter 15).

Generalized epilepsies, idiopathic

1. *Benign neonatal familial convulsions.* These patients are rare, and have clonic or apneic seizures in the first few days of life. Epilepsy is a sequela in a small percentage of affected patients.
2. *Benign neonatal convulsions.* These clonic or apneic seizures occur about the fifth day of life, but are benign and not followed either by epilepsy or by psychomotor slowing.
3. *Benign myoclonic epilepsy in infancy.* These patients have bursts of myoclonus in the first or second year of life; the EEG shows generalized spike-waves. Treatment is usually effective.
4. *Childhood absence epilepsy.* For description see Principle 21.
5. *Juvenile myoclonic epilepsy.* For description see Principle 23.
6. *Epilepsy with grand mal seizures on awakening.* This syndrome typically occurs between ten and twenty years, and a genetic predisposition is common.

Generalized epilepsies, cryptogenic or symptomatic

1. *West syndrome* (infantile spasms). For description see Principle 24.
2. *Lennox–Gastaut syndrome.* For description see Principle 25.
3. *Epilepsy with myoclonic-astatic seizures.* This subdivision may be a mild form of the Lennox–Gastaut syndrome. Heredity may play a role.
4. *Epilepsy with myoclonic absences.* This rare form of absence epilepsy is characterized by severe bilateral jerking and a relatively poor prognosis.

Generalized epilepsies, symptomatic

1. *Early myoclonic encephalopathy.* This poorly defined syndrome has its onset before three months; the prognosis is poor.
2. *Early infantile epileptic encephalopathy with suppression burst.* A serious syndrome, with early tonic seizures and frequent progression to West syndrome by four to six months.

Uncertain – either partial or generalized epilepsies

1. *Neonatal seizures.* For description see Principle 11.
2. *Severe myoclonic epilepsy of infancy.* A syndrome of early normal development followed by treatment resistant seizures of various types and by psychomotor retardation.
3. *Epilepsy with continuous spike-waves during slow wave sleep.* Generalized tonic–clonic seizures are typical in these patients who have an epileptic pattern during slow wave sleep.
4. *Acquired epileptic aphasia* (Landau–Kleffner syndrome). This syndrome in childhood is characterized by an acquired aphasia and multifocal EEG spikes and spike-waves. Epileptic seizures and psychomotor disturbances occur in two-thirds of patients.

Special epileptic syndromes

1. *Febrile convulsions.* For description see Principle 38.
2. *Single seizures.* For description see Principle 43.
3. *Seizures occurring only in response to an acute metabolic or toxic event.*

Unfortunately, it is not always possible to classify a patient into an epilepsy syndrome, just as the etiology of the epilepsy may remain elusive. It is almost always possible, however, to classify the patient's seizures; seizure classification is discussed in the next principle.

---

13 Virtually all seizures can be classified as either partial or generalized

---

Although modification and improvement of the classification of epileptic syndromes continues, the classification of epileptic seizures is more advanced. Even though the seizure diagnosis is a highly empirical method of determining therapy, and in spite of the limited theoretical basis for its use, it seems likely that this diagnostic approach will long remain valid. The reasons for the continuing dominance of the seizure diagnosis are twofold. First, epilepsy apparently has several mechanisms, and it is likely that each mechanism relates to only one or two of the various seizure types presently described. Second, an understanding of the basic mechanisms of the epilepsies that would have clear-cut therapeutic implications still seems a distant ideal. For the foreseeable future, therefore, the seizure type is the best information on which to base a therapeutic decision for the symptomatic treatment of epilepsy.

The first international classification of epileptic seizures (Gastaut, 1970) was the product of many years of effort by a group of experts. It proved very useful, but important refinements were afforded in 1981 by the use of videotape data (Commission on Classification and Terminology of the International League Against Epilepsy, 1981).

Seizures are fundamentally divided into two groups – partial and generalized. Partial seizures have clinical or electroencephalographic evidence of a local onset, but the word partial does not imply a highly discrete focus; such a focus often does not exist. The abnormal discharge usually arises in a portion of one hemisphere and may spread to other parts of the brain during a seizure. Generalized seizures, however, have no evidence of localized onset – the clinical manifestations and abnormal electrical discharge give no clue to the locus of onset of the abnormality, if indeed such a locus exists.

Partial seizures are divided into three groups: (1) simple partial seizures, (2) complex partial seizures, and (3) partial seizures which secondarily generalize. Simple partial seizures (SP) are associated with preservation of consciousness and unilateral hemispheric involvement. Complex partial seizures (CP) are associated with alteration or loss of consciousness and bilateral hemispheric involvement (for exceptions see Principles 16 and 17). A partial seizure secondarily generalized is a generalized tonic–clonic (GTC) seizure that proceeds directly from either a simple partial seizure or a complex partial seizure (Principle 20).

The distinction between simple partial seizures and complex partial seizures is clarified by the observation that neurologic insults that are confined to one hemisphere, such as a unilateral cerebral stroke, generally spare consciousness, whereas bilateral cerebral (or brain stem) involvement causes alteration of consciousness.

Consciousness in this context is defined as responsiveness. If the patient has some decrement in ability to respond to exogenous stimuli, then responsiveness, and therefore consciousness, is considered to be altered or lost. Obviously, the degree of difficulty of the task presented will, in part, affect the application of this definition to an individual patient. Exceptional patients with discrete lesions may be unresponsive but aware (e.g., with aphasia); in these patients, whose recall of ictal events is normal, consciousness is considered to be intact. Although responsiveness clearly represents a limited view of consciousness, this working definition allows clinical utilization of the classification of epileptic seizures, since the ability to respond during a seizure can usually be tested.

PRINCIPLE 13

One of the problems with the earlier international classification of epileptic seizures was its failure to provide for seizure progression. The 1981 classification provides, for partial seizures, for example, six possible progressions:

1. A simple partial seizure may exist alone (with preservation of consciousness).
2. A simple partial seizure may progress to a complex partial seizure (with alteration of consciousness).
3. A complex partial seizure may exist alone (with alteration of consciousness at onset).
4. A simple partial seizure may progress to a generalized tonic–clonic seizure (with alteration of consciousness).
5. A complex partial seizure may progress to a generalized tonic–clonic seizure (with alteration of consciousness at onset).
6. A simple partial seizure may progress to a complex partial seizure, which may then progress to a generalized tonic–clonic seizure (with alteration of consciousness).

These possibilities are summarized in Table 13.1. In patients with partial seizures, this classification is easily applied clinically to the patient's history. If consciousness is preserved throughout the attack, then the seizure is termed simple partial. If consciousness is lost at the onset, then the attack is a complex partial seizure; if the complex partial seizure is preceded by an aura, then the complex partial seizure has a simple partial onset. Any attack may, on occasion, progress to a generalized tonic–clonic seizure.

If there is no evidence of localized onset, then the attack is a generalized seizure. As heterogeneous as the partial seizures are, the generalized seizures are more so. The generalized seizures include (1) generalized tonic–clonic seizures (grand mal), (2) absence seizures (petit mal), (3) myoclonic seizures, (4) atonic seizures, (5) clonic seizures, and (6) tonic seizures. These seizures are listed in descending frequency of occurrence in the average mixed population of epileptic children and adults. Each of these types will be discussed in Chapter 5.

Table 13.1 Possible progression of partial seizures

Seizure progression	Seizure name
SP	Simple partial seizure
SP → CP	Complex partial seizure (with SP onset)
CP	Complex partial seizure
SP → GTC	Partial seizures secondarily generalized – generalized tonic–clonic seizure
CP → GTC	Partial seizures secondarily generalized – generalized tonic–clonic seizures
SP → CP → GTC	Partial seizures secondarily generalized – generalized tonic–clonic seizures

14 Most patients have a limited variety of seizure types

It is not true that most patients suffer a wide variety of seizure types. In fact, most patients have relatively stereotyped seizure patterns, and careful history-taking will usually reveal the pattern. The absence seizure pattern, for example, remains relatively constant in an individual patient, even though it is hetero-geneous among patients (Penry et al., 1975). In any patient with absence seizures, much of the variability in seizure pattern is clearly related to the patient's environment; these differences in seizure pattern, therefore, are not indicative of some new, fundamental alteration in the pattern of the abnormal electrical discharge.

The recognition of seizure progression is necessary for appropriate grouping of the seizure types. Upon questioning a patient about the nature of his attacks, it is common to discover that what at first appear to be several different types of seizures are in fact fragments (or variants) of a single seizure type. A good medical history will establish the possible progression of one kind of attack to another; a single type of attack may appear to be a variety of attacks to the patient because of its fragmented presentation and because different fragments of the seizure occur at different times.

Although most patients have a basic seizure type, with variations, a few will have a genuinely wide repertory of attacks. For example, the Lennox–Gastaut syndrome (Principle 25) is characterized by a variety of seizures in an individual patient. A carefully taken history, however, will usually allow grouping of the seizures into only two or three types. Another exception to the limited variety in seizure types occurs in the many patients who have generalized tonic–clonic seizures in addition to their fundamental seizure type. These generalized tonic–clonic seizures are often secondary to the fundamental seizure type (Principle 20); they are obviously classified separately and are usually treated differently.

15 Precipitation of epileptic seizures is influenced by the type of epileptic syndrome, patient variability, and environmental factors

Each epileptic syndrome is characterized by its own susceptibility to seizure pre-cipitation. Individual patients, of course, also vary widely in their susceptibility to seizure induction. Some patients have seizures only with major provocation; others have seizures with the slightest precipitating factor and still others have spontaneous seizures. Superimposed on this heterogeneity of syndromes and patients are the many factors that can induce a seizure. The precipitation of seizures can occur in a very nonspecific manner, or it can be specific, responding only to highly circumscribed stimuli. In absence epilepsy, patients frequently have seizures in response to hyperventilation – a good example of nonspecific seizure induction; a different, but overlapping, subset of absence patients will have seizures with photic stimulation. Patients with certain musicogenic epilepsies, on the other hand, have seizures induced only by very specific musical sounds.

Figures 15.1 and 15.2 are adapted from Engel (1989), and pictorially describe seizure susceptibility from the standpoint of the nonepileptic person (a person with no evidence of a seizure disorder), the nonepileptic person stressed by the environment, the person with epilepsy, and the person with epilepsy when stressed by the environment. The environmental factors considered are often under the patient's control.

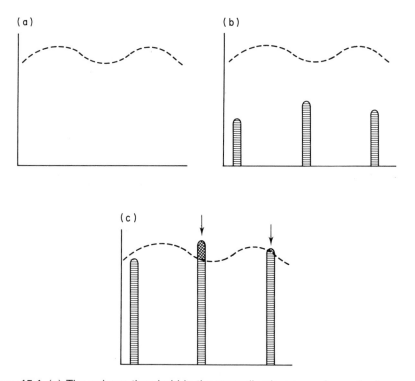

Figure 15.1 (a) The seizure threshold in the nonepileptic person (wavy line). Although no documentation exists for the variation – over time – of this threshold, such is assumed to be present. (b) Environmental factors (tall spikes) in the nonepileptic person do not reach threshold; seizures do not occur. (c) Environmental factors in the nonepileptic person are now more prominent, and on two occasions seizures (arrows) occur as threshold is exceeded. (Modified from Engel, 1989.)

PRINCIPLE 15

(a)

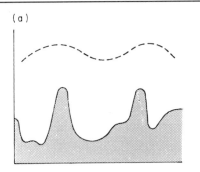

(b)

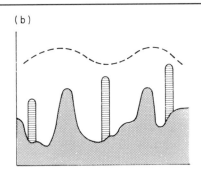

(c)

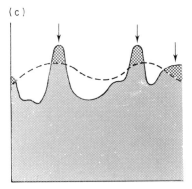

(d)

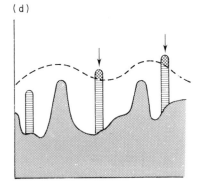

(e)

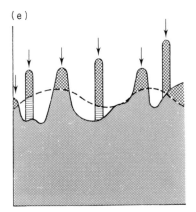

Figure 15.2 (a) Epileptic diathesis (dark portion) is also assumed to vary with time. The diathesis shortens the distance from the normal baseline (wavy line). Seizures are more likely but do not occur in this figure. (b) Environmental stresses (tall spikes) are added to the epileptic diathesis, but still seizures do not occur. (c) Seizures (arrows) occur as the epileptic disorder is out of control. (d) Seizures occur in predisposed patient, but only with environmental stress. (e) Seizures occur both because of the epileptic disorder and because of environmental factors. (Modified from Engel, 1989.)

Figure 15.1(a) shows the fluctuating seizure threshold of the nonepileptic person; everyone has a potential threshold and everyone is at risk for seizures (Principle 9). In the nonepileptic person this threshold is high. Usually, as shown in Figure 15.1(b), stresses experienced by nonepileptic persons do not cause seizures. These stresses vary widely and include such events as sleep deprivation, alcohol withdrawal, head injury, or even meningitis. In Figure 15.1(c), the environmental stresses overcome the normal threshold and seizures occur. Some – but not all – persons in this category will develop chronic seizures – epilepsy.

In Figure 15.2(a), a person with epilepsy has a decrease in threshold – a shortening of the safety margin for the likelihood of a seizure. No seizure occurs, however, because the threshold is not exceeded and no environmental stress factors are present. In 15.2(b), environmental factors and stresses are superimposed on the epileptic diathesis, but again the seizure threshold is not exceeded. Appropriate antiepileptic drug therapy may maintain this margin in favor of the patient. Seizures occur in epileptic persons in Figures 15.2(c), 15.2(d), and 15.2(e). In Figure 15.2(c), the epileptic predisposition itself is out of control and seizures occur at irregular intervals (intervals which, incidentally, are usually quite inexplicable). Additional medications may – or may not – cause a reversion to Figure 15.2(a), where control is maintained. In Figure 15.2(d), the epileptic diathesis is fundamentally controlled, but precipitating factors such as sleep deprivation – in the predisposed person – cause seizures at specific moments, often correlated with the environmental events. Figure 15.2(e) demonstrates the worst possible scenario: the patient has seizures both from the epileptic predisposition and from environmental factors. A patient in this last category might, for example, have partial epilepsy, fail to comply with the appropriate antiepileptic drug regimen, and superimpose sleep deprivation on this noncompliance. Status epilepticus may occur.

Most common nonspecific stimuli have been noted above. Specific stimuli have been extensively reviewed (Forster and Booker, 1984); the variability of such stimuli is quite remarkable but will not be further considered here.

4 Diagnosis: Partial Seizures

> **16** Simple partial seizures are not associated with loss of consciousness

Simple partial seizures are the most localized of the partial seizures. The discharge is usually confined to a single hemisphere, and the symptoms are specific to the affected brain region. It is the failure of the discharge to spread throughout the brain that explains the sparing of consciousness (see Principle 17 for the definition of consciousness).

The current international classification of seizures (Commission on Classification and Terminology of the International League Against Epilepsy, 1981) lists four main groups of simple partial seizures: (1) simple partial seizures with motor signs, (2) simple partial seizures with sensory symptoms, (3) simple partial seizures with autonomic symptoms or signs, and (4) simple partial seizures with psychic symptoms. The seizures in Group 1, focal motor attacks (e.g., clonic jerking of an arm), and Group 2, focal sensory attacks (e.g., the sensation of foul odor or taste), are the most commonly observed types.

An aura is nothing more than a simple partial seizure. The word aura (from the Greek, meaning 'breeze') traditionally has been used in epilepsy to refer to the onset of a seizure which the patient is able to describe because he is conscious during the event. The seizure that follows the aura, again from tradition, is usually associated with alteration of consciousness and is usually a complex partial or generalized tonic–clonic seizure. There is nothing fundamentally erroneous about this description, but a broader view is useful. First, the aura often does not progress further; the aura itself is the seizure. It is the reflection of abnormal neuronal discharge as perceived by the patient. Second, since consciousness is preserved during an aura, and since only a portion of the brain is involved, the attack is, by definition, a simple partial seizure. Any partial seizure may progress to another seizure type, and an aura is just one kind of simple partial seizure. A simple partial seizure may precede either a complex partial seizure or a generalized tonic–clonic seizure (see Table 13.1). This progression is apparent to those who treat many patients with partial seizures; treatment often decreases the frequency of the secondary attacks but leaves the patient with the simple partial seizures (auras).

A special type of simple partial seizure with motor signs is that in which spread occurs 'to contiguous cortical areas producing a sequential involvement of body parts in an epileptic march' (Commission on Classification and Terminology of the International League Against Epilepsy, 1981). Hughlings Jackson contributed to the understanding of such seizures and referred to them as 'cortical epilepsy'. Charcot, however, is credited with popularizing the term 'Jacksonian seizure' for the simple partial motor seizure which 'marches' along the cortex and body parts (Kelly, 1939).

The occurrence of psychic symptoms as the sole manifestation of a simple partial seizure is uncommon but noteworthy. For many years, any seizure characterized by higher cortical dysfunction was described as 'psychomotor' or 'temporal lobe', independent of the patient's state of consciousness. With video recording, it is clear that a few patients can have seizures characterized by paroxysmal symptoms such as *déjà vu*, forced thinking, or overwhelming fear, without alteration of consciousness. These attacks come from localized discharges and deserve to be called simple partial seizures; the 1981 classification of seizures allows for this rather unusual possibility. Overall, however, psychic symptoms are more commonly observed in complex partial seizures.

Although the vast majority of simple partial seizures have only unilateral hemispheric involvement, very rarely a simple partial seizure will involve *both* hemispheres simultaneously with sparing of consciousness (Weinberger and Lusins, 1973). These seizures apparently occur because of an abnormal bilateral discharge of limited extent. An actual recorded example documented a patient who had twitching of the left face and right arm simultaneously, with normal communication during the attack. One might call such an attack a 'bilateral simple partial seizure.'

The prognosis of simple partial seizures is exceedingly variable and is mostly dependent on the etiology. A small cortical venous malformation that causes contralateral focal motor signs may be surgically correctable with minimal deficit. A gustatory or olfactory simple partial seizure is sometimes a premonitory sign of a glioma (not always, as shown by Howe and Gibson, 1982); the prognosis may be poor. Some patients have continuous simple partial seizures (epilepsia partialis continua), which are often unresponsive to either medical or surgical therapy.

One subgroup of simple partial seizures occurs in the syndrome *benign childhood epilepsy with centrotemporal spikes*; this entity is also called 'sylvian seizures' (Lombroso, 1967) or 'rolandic epilepsy'. According to Loiseau and Duche (1989), the syndrome is defined by five major characteristics: (1) the age of onset is between two and thirteen, (2) it occurs in otherwise normal children having no neurologic or intellectual deficit, (3) in most cases, the seizures are partial with motor signs – although frequently associated with somatosensory symptoms; the attacks are sleep-related in 75% of patients, (4) the interictal EEG demonstrates a spike focus located in the centrotemporal (rolandic) area; the EEG background is normal, and (5) spontaneous remission occurs during adolescence. Others have noted a favorable prognosis with or without treatment (Beaussart and Faou,

1978). The seizures are most often characterized by orofacial and oropharyngeal involvement with either somatosensory symptoms or clonic jerking; both secondary generalization (Loiseau and Duche, 1989) and partial status epilepticus may occur (Fejerman and Di Blasi, 1987). When treated, the seizures are usually easily controlled (Holmes, 1992).

Simple partial seizures are surprisingly difficult to record electrographically. In one series, scalp electrodes were effective in recording only 10% of the attacks, whereas subdural electrodes detected almost 90% of the simple partial seizures in the same patient group (Devinsky et al., 1989a).

The temporary weakness or paralysis (Todd's paralysis) that sometimes follows simple partial seizures is more likely to be caused by active inhibition of neuronal function than by 'neuronal exhaustion'; in this regard one cannot discern ictal from postictal paralysis with any certainty (Efron, 1961).

---

17 Complex partial seizures are always associated with loss of consciousness

---

Complex partial seizures are the most common refractory seizure type in adults. The seizure begins as a localized discharge, but in cases where consciousness is lost at the onset of the attack (i.e., not preceded by a simple partial seizure), bilateral hemispheric involvement occurs extremely rapidly. Complex partial seizures have, in the past, been called temporal lobe seizures or psychomotor seizures. The discharges arise in one temporal lobe in most patients; others have discharges which arise from the frontal lobe or other areas. Even though the psyche is always involved, not all such seizures have motor manifestations. Automatisms may occur in complex (but not simple) partial seizures (Principle 18). A complex partial seizure may begin with alteration of consciousness or it may be preceded by a simple partial seizure (aura); it may be followed by a secondarily generalized tonic–clonic seizure (Table 13.1).

There is some important dissent regarding the thesis that bilateral hemispheric involvement is necessary for alteration of consciousness. Gloor et al. (1980) evaluated 69 complex partial seizures and found 'no evidence for bilateral spread' of the discharge in 19, using depth EEG recordings. They concluded that 'bilateral spread is not a necessary prerequisite for the occurrence of loss of consciousness'. They noted, however, that bilateral spread is the most common feature seen with loss of consciousness and that the mechanism of unilaterally induced loss of consciousness is unknown. This sophisticated study attempted to prove the nonexistence of an electrical discharge in part of the brain by inference from depth electrode recordings; the degree of uncertainty attached to such inferences is unknown, especially in view of the limitations of depth electrodes in detecting distant generators (Gloor, 1984).

Other characteristics of complex partial seizures have been described by Theodore *et al.* (1983a), who found that the duration of the attacks in their patients ranged from 11 seconds to almost 8 minutes (mean, 2 minutes). Automatisms occurred in 96% of the seizures. Only seven seizures were preceded by auras. Escueta *et al.* (1977) studied 76 seizures in 14 patients; there were two groups: (1) patients with an initial motionless stare, and (2) patients with automatisms at the onset of the seizure. The latter group may be less responsive to temporal lobectomy, as these investigators noted in a further study of 691 complex partial seizures in 79 patients (Delgado-Escueta *et al.*, 1981a).

The correct diagnosis of complex partial seizures of frontal lobe origin is of special interest, considering the frequent confusion of these seizures with psychogenic attacks (Williamson, 1992). On occasion, these seizures will be short, with minimal postictal abnormality; bizarre automatisms may also be present.

Differentiation of transient cerebral ischemia from simple partial seizures is usually not difficult; when consciousness is altered during the attack, however, the differential diagnosis between cerebral ischemia and complex partial seizures may not be easy. The former usually occur in older, susceptible persons, and repeated attacks may produce a persistent deficit; most seizures do not produce a lasting deficit. The duration of the attack may be the most useful differentiating feature: transient ischemia usually lasts longer than most seizures.

The prognosis for seizure control in patients with complex partial seizures is often poor, even in patients whose etiologic diagnosis appears not to be life threatening. Better medical and surgical therapies are greatly needed for this seizure type.

---

18 By definition, epileptic automatisms can only occur when consciousness is altered

Automatisms are highly integrated, complex behavioral acts occurring during seizures, of which the patient has no recollection and during which responsiveness is altered (Principle 13). Another term for automatisms is automatic behavior. Automatisms include lip smacking, fumbling of the hands, shuffling of the feet, and walking. Although a dissenting view is held by Munari and Bancaud (1985), most authorities consider that automatisms can only occur, by definition, during altered consciousness. Therefore, any act occurring during an epileptic seizure that requires integration of high-level cortical function may be considered automatic, provided that consciousness is altered. The automatisms of frontal lobe origin appear to be the most bizarre; kicking, thrashing, sexual motions, and vocalization are often observed (Williamson *et al.*, 1985) and can be mistakenly diagnosed as psychogenic.

Automatisms are relatively nonspecific; they occur in both generalized seizures and partial seizures and are apparently determined as much by influences outside the brain as by those within the brain. The nature of the automatism is often determined, therefore, by the patient's environment, either internal or external. A highly detailed classification of automatisms may be found in the work by Penry and Dreifuss (1969); this classification can be simplified into three subgroups:

1. *De novo automatisms from internal stimuli* (including 'release' phenomena), for example, chewing, lip smacking, swallowing, scratching, rubbing, picking, fumbling, running, and disrobing.
2. *De novo automatisms from external stimuli*, for example, responding to pin prick, drinking from a cup, chewing gum placed in the mouth, and pushing in response to restraint.
3. *Perseverative automatisms* (the continuation of any complex act initiated prior to loss of consciousness), for example, chewing food, using fork or spoon, drinking, and walking.

Automatisms may occur in generalized seizures as well as in partial seizures. Automatisms are so common in absence seizures, for example, that any seizure longer than 7 seconds has more than a 50% chance of having associated automatisms; a seizure longer than 18 seconds has a 95% chance of associated automatisms (Penry *et al.*, 1975). The commonly occurring automatisms in absence seizures are much the same as in complex partial seizures, although they are usually somewhat less complicated or prolonged. Lip smacking, chewing, and fumbling of the fingers are commonly observed in absence seizures; less common are swallowing, lip licking, grimacing, yawning, scratching, rubbing, shuffling the legs, walking, and stepping in place. In 374 video-analyzed seizures, automatisms were noted in 236 (63%); almost 90% of patients showed automatisms in at least one attack (Penry *et al.*, 1975). In the study by Holmes *et al.* (1987) automatisms were found in 44% of typical absence seizures and 22% of atypical absence seizures; this difference was statistically significant.

Whether the observed automatisms are ictal or postictal can, in some seizures, be difficult to determine. In absence seizures, all automatisms are ictal because there is no abnormal postictal state. In complex partial seizures, both ictal and postictal automatisms may be observed, but the exact onset of the postictal state itself may be difficult to define. Extensive data are available on the nature of automatisms in absence seizures (Penry *et al.*, 1975) and complex partial seizures (Escueta *et al.*, 1977; Theodore *et al.*, 1983a; Williamson *et al.*, 1985). The data are probably more complete for absence seizures (Principle 21) than for the relatively heterogeneous complex partial seizures (Principle 17). The full spectrum of the latter includes such characteristics as formed hallucinations, illusions, affective symptoms, and cognitive symptoms (all during altered consciousness);

PRINCIPLE 18

these have been well reviewed by Daly (1975). The relationship of violent behavior to epilepsy, especially complex partial seizures, is discussed in Principle 37.

---

19 Psychic phenomena may not be helpful in the diagnosis of epilepsy

---

Hughlings Jackson (1888) wrote prolifically about alterations of consciousness, especially about partial alterations in epileptic patients who had psychic phenomena during their attacks. He was fully cognizant, however, of the pitfalls of overdiagnosing epilepsy from such data, as he wrote: 'I should never. . .diagnose epilepsy from the paroxysmal occurrence of "reminiscence" without other symptoms, although I should suspect epilepsy, if that super-positive mental state began to occur very frequently. . . '. Nevertheless, a tendency remains to consider such phenomena as *déjà vu* as highly suggestive of an epileptic discharge. Harper and Roth (1962) evaluated the frequency of 'temporal lobe' symptomatology in 30 patients with phobic-anxiety (Principle 34) and compared the occurrence of these symptoms to that in 30 patients with complex partial seizures. The results are shown in Table 19.1.

Notable is the observation that the symptoms of derealization and 'loss of feeling of familiarity' are actually more common in the phobic-anxiety syndrome

Table 19.1 'Temporal lobe' symptomology in epileptic and nonepileptic patients

	Phobic anxiety syndrome	Complex partial seizures	Statistical difference
Depersonalization	17	11	NS
Derealization	11	0	$p < 0.01$
Loss of feeling of familiarity (*jamais vu*)	9	1	$p < 0.02$
Déjà vu sensation	12	7	NS
Formed hallucinations (visual, auditory, olfactory)	11	4	NS
Illusions and distortions of perception, including body image changes	12	7	NS
Idea of a 'presence'	14	7	NS

Modified from Harper and Roth (1962).
NS, Not significant.

than in patients with complex partial seizures (termed 'temporal lobe epilepsy' by the authors, usage consistent with the date of publication). None of the above symptoms, so often thought to be characteristic of complex partial seizures, are more common in patients with epilepsy than in patients with psychiatric problems. The diagnostic value of such phenomena are, therefore, clearly in doubt. When such a symptom is indeed epileptic and consciousness is preserved during the symptom, the attacks are best classified as simple partial seizures to designate the localized nature of the abnormal discharge (Principle 16).

Certain criteria may help establish which phenomena are epileptic. Sensations tend to be more vivid, more stable, and more stereotyped in patients with epilepsy. Although short, paroxysmal symptoms were noted in Harper and Roth's study – in both the phobic-anxiety group and the epileptic group – psychic phenomena were usually long lasting in the phobic group but not in the epileptic group; the occurrence of such symptoms for many minutes or even hours suggested that the symptoms were not epileptic in nature. Often, patients with epilepsy had their psychic symptoms only in association with other epileptic phenomena, such as strange feelings in the stomach (Harper and Roth, 1962).

In summary, the use of psychic symptoms to support the diagnosis of epilepsy is often inappropriate; in virtually all patients other corroborative data are essential to the establishment of the diagnosis.

5 Diagnosis: Generalized Seizures

---

20 Most generalized tonic–clonic (grand mal) seizures are secondary to another seizure type

---

The prevalence of *primary* generalized tonic–clonic seizures, has been overemphasized. In fact, most generalized tonic–clonic seizures occur secondarily to a less dramatic seizure type. Video recordings of secondary generalized tonic–clonic seizures abound, but, recordings of primary generalized tonic–clonic seizures are relatively uncommon; such primary attacks are probably most common in drug (including alcohol) withdrawal. Frequently one elicits a medical history of the progression of partial seizures to generalized tonic–clonic seizures (Principle 13); when generalized tonic–clonic attacks occur in patients with partial epilepsy, most – if not all – such attacks are secondarily induced. In generalized seizures (other than the generalized tonic–clonic seizure itself), similar observations can be confirmed. For example, progression of absence seizures to generalized tonic–clonic seizures has been documented clinically and electrographically (Oller-Daurella, 1974; Niedermeyer, 1976; Theodore *et al.*, 1994b), and progression of clonic seizures to generalized tonic–clonic seizures has been noted (Porter and Sato, 1982; Theodore *et al.*, 1994b).

Since seizures of both the partial and the generalized categories can progress to generalized tonic–clonic seizures, the latter appear to be a stereotyped expression of maximal involvement of cerebral neurons; this would suggest that the generalized tonic–clonic seizure is the only seizure type worthy of the term 'generalized'. Other seizures in the so-called 'generalized' classification are not truly generalized in the sense of maximal neuronal involvement, but merely have submaximal bilateral brain involvement. This bilateral involvement, as seen in absence or clonic seizures, for example, may progress to maximal involvement, that is, to secondary generalized tonic–clonic seizures. Unfortunately, such progression was not recognized in the 1981 international classification of seizures; for consistency, this deficiency of the classification will be ignored here. Minor revision of the classification will eventually be necessary to account for this progression.

PRINCIPLE 20

From the foregoing discussion, it is obviously necessary, in patients with generalized tonic–clonic seizures, to establish the nature of any other seizure type at the time of the initial and subsequent evaluations; appropriate therapy can then be instituted for the fundamental seizure type as well as for the tonic–clonic seizures. The stereotyped nature of generalized tonic–clonic seizures as compared with other seizure types makes them relatively easy to distinguish by history. Other seizure types are more subtle and are often more heterogeneous. When taking the medical history, first establish whether or not generalized tonic–clonic seizures are present and are not, for example, psychogenic attacks; then search for a history of other seizure types.

The generalized tonic–clonic seizure is not a random flailing of the body and limbs but a describable, circumscribed event. Theodore *et al.* (1994b) studied 120 spontaneous generalized tonic–clonic seizures in 47 patients with video-EEG telemetry recordings; most of these seizures were secondarily generalized, reflecting the hospital-based population. The mean duration of the seizures was 62 seconds; the longest was only 108 seconds and the shortest 16 seconds. Although the seizures were heterogeneous, the attacks could be divided into seven phases, beginning with the antecedent seizure and ending with the clonic phase (Table 20.1). Every seizure had either a tonic or a clonic phase, but both are not necessarily present in all seizures.

Isolated fragments of such seizures are frequent (Principle 14). The fragments may be the result of partially effective antiepileptic drug treatment, and either tonic or clonic motions may be observed. When the complete attack occurs, it is well described by Gastaut and Broughton (1972); Tables 20.2 and 20.3 summarize their observations.

In addition to the above sequence of events, autonomic changes are prominent. The heart rate and blood pressure may double, and the bladder pressure may increase up to sixfold. Pupillary mydriasis and glandular hypersecretion of the

---

Table 20.1 The seven phases of the secondarily generalized tonic–clonic seizure (GTCS)

A. The antecedent seizure (which precedes the GTCS itself)
    Phase I: The simple partial seizure
    Phase II: One of four seizure types:
                  (1) Complex partial seizure (may follow Phase I)
                  (2) Clonic seizure
                  (3) Tonic seizure
                  (4) Absence seizure

B. The generalized tonic–clonic seizure
    Phase III: Onset of generalization (e.g., versive head motion)
    Phase IV: Pre-tonic clonic phase
    Phase V: Tonic phase
    Phase VI: Tremulousness phase (onset of clonic)
    Phase VII: Clonic phase

Table 20.2 Tonic phase of generalized tonic–clonic seizures

1. Usually lasts 10–20 seconds
2. Begins with brief *flexion*:
    (a)   muscles contract
    (b)   the eyelids open; eyes look up
    (c)   the arms are elevated, abducted, and externally rotated; elbows are semiflexed
    (d)   the legs are less involved, but may be flexed
3. *Extension* phase is more prolonged:
    (a)   involves first the back and neck
    (b)   a tonic cry may occur – lasts 2–12 seconds
    (c)   the arms extend
    (d)   legs are extended, adducted, and externally rotated
4. The *tremor* begins:
    (a)   the tremor is a repetitive relaxation of the tonic contraction
    (b)   starts at 8 per second, gradually coarsens to 4 per second
    (c)   leads to the clonic phase

From Gastaut and Broughton (1972), courtesy of Charles C. Thomas, Publisher, Springfield, Illinois.

Table 20.3 Clonic phase of generalized tonic–clonic seizures

1. Usually lasts about 30 seconds
2. Begins when the muscular relaxations completely interrupt the tonic contraction
3. Brief, violent flexor spasms of the whole body
4. The tongue is often bitten

From Gastaut and Broughton (1972), courtesy of Charles C. Thomas, Publisher, Springfield, Illinois.

skin and salivary glands occur. Cyanosis of the skin is correlated with the accompanying apnea (Gastaut and Broughton, 1972).

The EEG accompaniments of the generalized tonic–clonic seizure are dramatic but often obscured by muscle artifact. The initial EEG change is usually a desynchronization lasting 1 to 3 seconds, followed by 10 seconds of 10-Hz spikes; as the clonic phase predominates, the spikes are mixed with slow waves, and finally become a polyspike-and-wave pattern. The EEG is flat, or nearly flat, after a severe generalized tonic–clonic seizure but gradually recovers to normal rhythms.

The prognosis of generalized tonic–clonic seizures depends on the nature of the epileptic syndrome in question, which encompasses the etiology of the epilepsy and the other seizure types involved. In a few patients with only idiopathic generalized tonic–clonic seizures, the attacks may prove difficult to control.

The phases outlined in Table 20.1 are taken from the 120 seizures analyzed by Theodore *et al.* (1994b). Not all seizures had all phases. For example, 30 seizures had Phase I (simple partial onset) but 85 seizures began with Phase II (70 with complex partial). Of the 30 beginning with Phase I, 17 progressed through a complex partial seizure (Phase II) to the GTCS. Only 15 seizures began with a generalized seizure in Phase II (tonic 7, clonic 7, absence 1). Five GTCS were primarily generalized and had no antecedent seizure.

---

21 Absence seizures are well described despite their heterogeneity

Until the last decade, empirical descriptions of the various seizure types were quite inadequate, and our knowledge of exactly what typifies the various attacks was largely anecdotal. This inadequacy remains for rare seizure types.

The absence (petit mal) seizure was among the first to be adequately described (Penry et al., 1975) because of the high frequency of such attacks in affected children, techniques of intensive monitoring, and an outstanding population of such patients gathered by Dr F.E. Dreifuss at the University of Virginia. Absence epilepsy begins in childhood or early adolescence. Although absence seizures are virtually never reported as beginning after adolescence, certain forms of petit mal status apparently occur in later years as the presenting epileptic symptom (Porter and Penry, 1983); see Principle 31.

Prior to the study by Penry and Dreifuss (1969), the absence seizure had been characterized as an attack with a blank stare, motionlessness and unresponsiveness. Although unresponsiveness is the rule, motionlessness occurs in less than 10% of absence attacks; in fact, many other phenomena may accompany such attacks (Penry et al., 1975). Absence seizures are generally brief, usually lasting less than 10 seconds and very rarely longer than 45 seconds. The attacks are not associated with auras, postictal abnormalities, hallucinations, formed speech, or other symptoms characteristic of partial seizures, generalized tonic–clonic seizures, or infantile spasms. In a video analysis of 374 recorded absence seizures, the attacks were found to be characterized by some combination of the features given in Table 21.1.

In an important study of 926 video-taped absence seizures by Holmes et al. (1987), the investigators differentiated between typical and atypical absence attacks. The patients with atypical attacks had a much higher likelihood of having developmental delay or retardation, other seizure types (other than partial seizures), and EEG's with interictal abnormalities. The differences between the seizures of each group are also noteworthy. Typical absence seizures are more likely to be characterized by automatisms and eye blinking, whereas atypical absence seizures are typified by more prominent increases or decreases in muscle

Table 21.1 Features of absence seizures

Feature	Percentage of seizures*
Automatisms	63%
Mild clonic motion (usually eyelids)	46%
Decreased postural tone (usually head nodding)	23%
Increased postural tone (usually arching of the back)	5%
Autonomic phenomena	?

*Many patients had more than one feature. From Penry et al. (1975), with permission of Oxford University Press.

tone. Atypical absence seizures were significantly longer than typical absence seizures. The onset and cessation were abrupt in each type and neither was useful in distinguishing between the two groups. Finally, the authors concluded that typical and atypical absence attacks are not discrete entities but form a continuum.

Sato et al. (1983) conducted a follow-up study of 83 patients with absence seizures. The follow-up period averaged 9.5 years after the initial visit. Multivariate analysis of selected prognostic factors showed that normal or above-average intelligence was the single most important prognostic factor. Other factors suggestive of a favorable outcome included normal neurologic examination, male sex, and lack of hyperventilation-induced spike-waves on the EEG; 90% of patients with three or four of these criteria had stopped having seizures at the time of follow-up.

Although absence seizures may occur in several types of epilepsy, the attacks are most commonly seen in one of two epileptic syndromes. *Childhood absence epilepsy* (pyknolepsy) has its onset between four and ten years, with a peak at six to seven years. The attacks may occur many times daily; associated generalized tonic–clonic seizures are common. *Juvenile absence epilepsy* has its onset somewhat later, and the seizures occur less frequently. In both syndromes, the response to therapy and the prognosis is typically very good (Commission on Classification and Terminology of the International League Against Epilepsy, 1989; Porter, 1993).

Two other characteristics of absence epilepsy are worthy of mention. First, localized interictal spikes are common in the EEG's of such patients. In the study by Holmes et al. (1987), 10 of 37 patients with *typical* absence seizures had interictal focal or multifocal spikes or sharp waves. Second, these patients do not develop partial seizures over time. In the study by Sato et al. (1983), none of the 83 patients developed partial seizures in the follow-up period, although 3 had partial seizures at the time of initial diagnosis.

---

22 Mistaking absence seizures for complex partial seizures is a serious diagnostic error leading to inappropriate therapy

---

Despite the apparent differences between absence seizures and complex partial seizures, these seizure types are sometimes confused. The usual error is to classify an absence seizure as a complex partial seizure, and then to treat the patient with carbamazepine, phenytoin or phenobarbital, which will control the concomitant generalized tonic–clonic seizures, if present, but will leave the absence seizures uncontrolled. The following example is typical:

A 24-year-old, right-handed man had an 11-year history of uncontrolled attacks characterized by decreased responsiveness lasting less than 10 seconds, followed by rapid return to normal consciousness; the attacks occurred many times daily. He also had generalized tonic–clonic seizures three or four times a month. He was taking phenytoin (400 mg/day) and primidone (1250 mg/day). The EEG showed bilaterally synchronous 2.5 to 3.5-Hz spike-and-wave discharges on a diffusely slow background. On reevaluation, a seizure diagnosis of absence seizures with occasional generalized tonic–clonic attacks was made. When the patient was started on valproate and the primidone was gradually discontinued, he became seizure free. He obtained a driver's license and is employed.

Proper seizure diagnosis is made on the basis of many differential features, but in this patient the most helpful clinical sign was the *absence of a postictal abnormality*. Confusion, lethargy, or malaise is the rule after most complex partial seizures, but such abnormalities are virtually never present after absence attacks. Occasional complex partial attacks may be followed by instant mental clarity, but the patient will almost always describe other, longer attacks *with* a postictal abnormality; this evidence allows the proper diagnosis. Except in the Lennox–Gastaut syndrome, the coexistence of absence seizures and complex partial seizures in the same patient is unusual (Principle 25). The therapy of these two seizure types is entirely different (Principles 51 and 73), as is the prognosis of the associated syndromes.

The coexistence of absence seizures with generalized tonic–clonic attacks is not unusual. One-third of all patients with absence seizures also have infrequent generalized tonic–clonic seizures. In the study by Penry *et al.* (1975), 16 of 48 intensively studied patients with absence seizures also reported having had generalized tonic–clonic attacks. According to Holmes *et al.* (1987), these attacks are much more likely to be present in patients with atypical rather than with typical absence seizures; only 19% of their patients with typical absence seizures had associated generalized tonic–clonic attacks whereas 96% of patients with atypical absence had this associated seizure type. It may well be that most of these generalized tonic–clonic seizures are secondary to the absence attacks, but conclusive supporting data are not yet available (Principle 20). The occurrence of generalized tonic–clonic seizures in a patient with absence attacks requires a different therapeutic approach from that needed in patients who have only absence seizures (Principle 74).

23　Juvenile myoclonic epilepsy is an important, benign myoclonic syndrome

---

The syndrome of juvenile myoclonic epilepsy is worthy of special note because of the initial fear that the patient may have a fatal disease. In contrast to Lafora body disease, it is a rewarding disorder to recognize and treat. Typically, a teenager or preadolescent child will have the onset of sudden, sometimes explosive, uncontrollable myoclonic jerks. The jerks will be embarrassing, more frequent in the morning or on arising from sleep, and bothersome at the table when eating. The attacks occasionally progress to generalized tonic–clonic seizures, which may follow directly from an especially severe series of clonic seizures; the tonic–clonic seizures are secondary to the clonic attacks (Principle 20). Mental retardation does not occur. Attacks worsen with anxiety, sudden stimuli, or sleeplessness. The EEG typically shows generalized polyspike and wave abnormalities; photic stimulation may elicit an attack. Valproate is generally considered the therapy of choice and is superior to phenytoin for this syndrome. The following is a typical case:

A 19-year-old woman reported a history of several kinds of attacks which had begun in adolescence. Sudden unprovoked jerks occurred about once per week, affecting her arms most strongly and occasionally causing her to drop a cup or glass. About twice per month she had episodes of anxiety, a feeling of 'going away' terror, loss of control, and a racing heart beat. The latter spells became more frequent during periods of stress and were particularly related to school work. Generalized tonic–clonic seizures occurred about twice a year. She had originally been diagnosed as having complex partial seizures with secondary generalization; she was treated with carbamazepine, which controlled the generalized tonic–clonic seizures but did not affect the anxiety spells or the myoclonic jerks. Video-EEG monitoring showed generalized irregular interictal discharges; no EEG change was observed during the anxiety attacks. Treatment with valproic acid and with intermittent benzodiazepines controlled her symptoms.

The largest study of this disorder is by Janz and Christian (1957), who described 47 patients with juvenile myoclonic epilepsy; they were thought to represent 3% to 4% of all epilepsy patients. The usual age at onset of the disorder was between 10 and 23 years, and all but two patients had occasional generalized tonic–clonic seizures in addition to the myoclonic attacks. In a later review, Janz (1985) considered the syndrome in detail and has termed it 'epilepsy with impulsive petit mal' because of its close relationship to absence epilepsy. The EEG abnormalities, for example, often cannot be distinguished from that of juvenile absence epilepsy.

New approaches to molecular genetics are being vigorously pursued in epilepsy, especially in this frequently inherited syndrome. Considerable evidence suggests that the genetic abnormality for juvenile myoclonic epilepsy may reside on chromosome number six (Greenberg and Delgado-Escueta, 1993).

---

24 Onset of spasms before one year of age is the rule in 90% of patients with infantile spasms

Infantile spasms was first classified as an epileptic syndrome (Commision on Classification and Terminology of the International League Against Epilepsy, 1981) rather than a seizure type, but more recent consideration (Commission on Pediatric Epilepsy of the International League Against Epilepsy, 1992) has led to a revised view, namely that infantile spasms is a special seizure type, often occurring in clusters, with involvement of the axial musculature. The patient is said to have 'West Syndrome' when infantile spasms are associated with an hypsarrhythmia.

Although their heterogeneity is extraordinary, the seizures are usually divided into three different clinical types. The following description of each type is taken from the 5,042 recorded seizures reported by Kellaway *et al.* (1979):

1. Flexor spasms are characterized by 'flexion of the neck, arms, and legs' with prominent contraction of the abdominal muscles to 'cause the torso to jackknife at the waist'. The arms are either abducted or adducted.
2. Extensor spasms are characterized by 'extension of the neck and trunk with extensor abduction or adduction of the arms, legs, or both'.
3. Mixed flexor–extensor spasms were the most common type, usually with flexion of the body and arms and extension of the legs.

Numerous synonyms have been created to describe these heterogeneous seizures, including, according to Lacy and Penry (1976), (1) massive myoclonic jerks, (2) lightning major spasms, (3) flexion spasms, (4) greeting spasms, (5) salaam spasms, (6) jackknife convulsions, (7) infantile myoclonic epilepsy, and (8) Blitz-Nick-Krampfe.

As with many other epileptic syndromes, West syndrome is caused by many diverse etiological processes. Lacy and Penry (1976) have identified the most common as (1) idiopathic (approximately 40% of the cases), (2) maternal uterine hemorrhage, (3) maternal toxemia, (4) hydrocephalus, (5) congenital CNS infections (e.g., toxoplasmosis, cytomegalovirus), (6) prematurity (?), (7) low birth weight (?), (8) Aicardi syndrome, (9) perinatal delivery difficulties, (10) kernicterus, (11) trauma, (12) meningitis or encephalitis, (13) immunizations (especially pertussis?), (14) tuberous sclerosis, (15) phenylketonuria and other amino acid abnormalities, (16) neonatal hypoglycemia, and (17) pyridoxine deficiency (?). In some patients, focal cortical dysplasia has been detected by high resolution MRI or positron emission tomography using 18F-fluorodeoxyglucose. Most such abnormalities have been found in the temporo-occipito-parietal cortex.

The onset is usually within the first six months of life. In the series reported by Charleton (1975), 96% occurred within the first year. As noted above, the attacks themselves often cluster; the child may have a series of many seizures followed by relative quiescence.

The classic EEG finding, hypsarrhythmia (from the Greek, meaning 'high rhythm'), is seen in most patients, although it is most typical only in the early stages of the disorder (Hrachovy, 1982). The abnormality is an interictal EEG pattern characterized by 'a mixture of high-amplitude spikes and slow waves of varying duration and location, occurring continuously or in bursts' (Commission on Pediatric Epilepsy of the International League Against Epilepsy, 1992). When the EEG becomes more organized, as it apparently does with the passage of time, it has been called 'modified hypsarrhythmia'. At least three subgroups of the EEG abnormality have been described (Hrachovy, 1982), but there is little evidence that such differentiation is useful in predicting the prognosis of the seizures or the associated mental subnormality (Charleton, 1975).

The underlying reason for the form of these seizures is unknown. It is intriguing to speculate that the central nervous system has, in its early developmental years, only a limited repertoire of clinical signs and symptoms, and that seizures occurring at this time are more limited in their variability of expression than is the case in adults. Such speculation helps to explain the diverse causes of the syndrome, although it sheds little light on the basic mechanisms of the disorder. The two cases reported by Hrachovy et al. (1987) are instructive in that each was caused by near-drowning in children ages 16 months and 31 months, with onset of spasms within a few months thereafter; the age of vulnerability may not be as narrow as has been previously thought.

The prognosis of patients with infantile spasms is poor, and all but 5% of patients with West syndrome will develop mental retardation (Farrell, 1993a). Of the 214 patients followed for at least 3 years by Riikonen (1982), 19.6% had died and only 12% had developed normally. Following cessation of the infantile spasms, more than half the survivors had seizures of a different type, usually partial seizures. The data of Glaze et al. (1988) are also pessimistic; only 3 of 64 patients had 'normal development or mild impairment'. Many patients progress to the Lennox–Gastaut syndrome (Principle 25). The treatment of infantile spasms is considered in Principle 80.

25 Lennox–Gastaut syndrome is not a seizure type

'A stare, a jerk, a fall – these represent three seizure phenomena which differ widely in appearance. . .' Thus did Lennox (1960) set forth his 'petit mal triad', in which he distinguished three different groups correlated with three different seizure types. The first group is 'pure petit mal' (a stare), which comprises 79% of the triad in Lennox's series, and correlates rather well with what we now call absence seizures (Principle 26). Lennox even observed the coexistence of mild clonic motion and automatic behavior with the stare in this seizure type. The second group, 'myoclonia' (a jerk), is admittedly heterogeneous. Lennox divided myoclonias into several subgroups: (1) myoclonic epilepsy, which very roughly correlates to juvenile myoclonic epilepsy of Janz (Principle 23); (2) massive myoclonic jerks, which correlate fairly well with what we now know as infantile spasms (Principle 24); (3) myoclonus epilepsy – the progressive syndromes of genetic etiology (Principle 27); (4) epilepsia partialis continua, now considered to be a form of continuous simple partial seizures; and (5) palatal myoclonus, a specific myoclonic disorder. Finally, the third group, 'astatic epilepsy' (a fall), correlates best with atonic seizures (Principle 26).

Lennox coincidentally made three generalizations about the triad as a whole: (1) the phenomena frequently coexist in individual patients, (2) spike-and-wave abnormalities accompany the attacks, and (3) affected patients have a different response to drugs than do patients with 'convulsions'.

The major difficulty in understanding the triad was related to Lennox's attempt to equate seizure types with epileptic syndromes. Failure to separate the two resulted in confusion for both investigators and practicing physicians. Ironically, the Lennox–Gastaut syndrome represents a synthesis of Lennox's first unifying observation, that is, that the stare, jerk, and fall frequently coexist in the same patient. This epileptic syndrome was well defined by Gastaut *et al.* (1966), who described a heterogeneous population of patients with absence, clonic, and atonic seizures. Synonyms of the epileptic syndrome include Lennox syndrome, akinetic petit mal, myoclonic-astatic petit mal, and petit mal variant epilepsy; occasionally the term 'minor motor seizures' is also used to describe the attacks in these patients (Principle 29).

The Lennox–Gastaut syndrome usually begins between the ages of one and six years, though rarely it may occur as late as ten years of age or older. It may develop in patients who have had infantile spasms, but more often occurs spontaneously. The etiologies are diverse. Most patients are mentally retarded. The most devastating seizures are atonic; the head may drop suddenly onto the breakfast table, or the patient may fall precipitously to the floor. Injuries to the face and teeth are common, and helmets are necessary to protect the head. The absence seizures are usually brief and atypical (Principle 21); more pronounced tone changes are common (Holmes *et al.*, 1987). Brief tonic seizures may also occur (Farrell, 1993a), and any of these attacks – tonic, atonic, or absence – may be accompanied by myoclonic jerks. In some cases, the patient appears to be thrown to the floor by the violence of the clonic jerks. The seizures are often severe and intractable. The EEG commonly demonstrates continuous spike-and-wave abnormalities, usually at a rate which is less than three per second, and the complexes are often irregular and asymmetrical; multifocal spikes are also common. As the patient gets older, complex partial and generalized tonic–clonic seizures may become predominant.

The etiologies of the syndrome are many, especially brain malformations, perinatal hypoxic–ischemic brain injury, encephalitis, meningitis, and tuberous sclerosis; perhaps as many as 30% are cryptogenic (Farrell, 1993b). Positron emission tomographic (PET) studies have suggested that this heterogeneous syndrome may be divisible into subtypes based on differential glucose metabolism (Chugani *et al.*, 1987). Other PET studies suggest that those patients with partial seizures must be evaluated separately (Theodore *et al.*, 1987c).

Some patients appear to have continuous seizures, without remission. One may speculate in these cases that the level of mental function may be due to inadequate numbers of normal neurons, or alternatively, that the available neurons are functioning poorly because of the widespread, continuous nature of the abnormal discharge. Both factors are likely to be present in most of these patients.

---

26 Not every seizure associated with decreased tone is properly classified as atonic

---

In almost 25% of absence seizures, the attacks are associated with some loss of body muscle tone (Principle 21). Other seizures, such as simple or complex partial attacks, may also be associated with decreased postural tone. None of these seizures is properly termed atonic. The term 'atonic seizure' is reserved for an especially refractory group of seizures characterized by sudden and precipitous loss of tone. Patients may fall to the floor, often with injury to their head, face, or teeth. During a meal, the patient's head may fall forward onto the plate. Helmets, which are a necessity for many of these patients, afford considerable protection, but contribute greatly to the social stigma of their epilepsy. Most patients with absence seizures or complex partial seizures do not require helmets because the loss of tone is more gradual – they stumble and stagger but seldom fall suddenly; in these attacks the seizure rarely begins with loss of tone. An atonic attack may or may not be followed by a postictal abnormality. Other seizure types are common in patients with atonic seizures.

In earlier publications on epilepsy a curious use of the term 'akinetic' (without motion) occurred; it came to be synonymous with 'atonic' (without tone). This terminology is especially prevalent in discussions of the Lennox–Gastaut syndrome (Principle 25). In the international classification of epileptic seizures (Commission on Classification and Terminology of the International League Against Epilepsy, 1981), reference to akinetic seizures has been deleted. There is no evidence for the existence of a separate seizure type characterized only by motionlessness. In fact, many seizure types are characterized by motionlessness, and akinesis is not unique to any group. The preferred term for prominent, sudden loss of tone is atonic. The term 'astatic' (with motion) is also no longer recommended.

---

27 Myoclonus is often a seizure component rather than an independent seizure type

---

'Myoclonus' and 'clonus' have been used in different ways, leading to considerable confusion. 'Epileptic myoclonus' (which has been used to suggest cortical origin or involvement) is also a confusing term, since similar clinical and physiologic phenomena may occur in patients with and without epilepsy. A simple definition was suggested by Marsden *et al.* (1982): 'muscle jerking, irregular or rhythmic, arising in the central nervous system', which sets myoclonus off from other movement disorders such as tic, chorea, or dystonia. 'Clonic' seizures have been defined in the International Classification of Seizures: they are generalized attacks which lack a tonic phase. Myoclonic jerks are short-duration and rapid if repetitive (Hallett, 1985).

Unfortunately, the pathophysiology may be as confusing as the terminology. The basic disturbance in myoclonus (whether or not associated with seizures) is hyperactivity of the motor system, which can occur at a cortical, subcortical, or spinal level (Halliday, 1967; Hallett, 1985). In myoclonus of cortical origin, stimulus-evoked clinical jerks and enlarged somatosensory evoked potentials suggest increased sensitivity of the afferent reflex arc; there is, however, evidence for increased activity in efferent pathways as well (Dawson, 1947; Sutton and Mayer, 1974). Some patients experience exacerbation of myoclonus during voluntary movements.

Several anatomic and physiologic classifications of myoclonus have been proposed (Halliday, 1967; Hallett, 1985). 'Pyramidal' or 'cortical reflex myoclonus' may resemble a fragmentary focal seizure. It can be multifocal, accentuated either by voluntary movement (action myoclonus) or by somatosensory stimulation (reflex myoclonus). 'Giant' somatosensory evoked potentials may be present. A cortical spike precedes the electromyogram (EMG) burst, which is usually less than 50 milliseconds long. Interhemispheric spread follows a somatotopic pattern (Brown et al., 1991), with synchronous muscle activation of agonist and antagonist muscles. Flash-evoked cortical myoclonus is associated with occipital spikes, but unlike photosensitive epilepsy, responds to dopaminergic agonists (Artieda and Obeso, 1993).

'Non-pyramidal' or 'reticular reflex' myoclonus usually involves many muscles simultaneously. Jerks may be induced by voluntary movement or sensory stimulation. Retrograde conduction from a site of origin in caudal brainstem reticular formation can involve cranial nerves (Zuckerman and Glaser, 1972). Cortical spikes are projected (and are not etiologic for the myoclonus); the SEP is not increased.

'Primary generalized epileptic myoclonus' usually is characterized by small focal jerks involving the fingers: minipolymyoclonus. Generalized, synchronous, whole body jerks arise from ascending subcortical impulses and may be preceded by slow frontocentral EEG negativity. Similar indistinguishable phenomena may occur in conditions such as motor neuron disease.

'Non-epileptic' (extra-cortical) myoclonus includes dystonic forms originating in the basal ganglia, segemental – including spinal and palatal myoclonus – and periodic movements of sleep. The EMG burst length is longer than in cortical myoclonus and there is no EEG correlate. Clinical features may mimic a cortical origin, and EEG back-averaging from the EMG may be necessary to make the distinction (Shibasaki and Kuroiwa, 1975). Palatal myoclonus has been reported in conjunction with more widespread epilepsia partialis continua (EPC) (Tatum et al., 1991). Psychogenic myoclonus can be segmental or generalized, is often related to stress, and may be associated with underlying psychopathology and other signs of functional neurologic illness (Monday and Janovic, 1993).

Myoclonic and clonic jerks can be seen in a wide range of neurological disorders; their value for differential diagnosis, therefore, is limited. Myoclonus may occur either alone, or accompanied by seizures, in a number of progressive or nonprogressive encephalopathies such as GM 2 gangliosidoses, subacute sclerosing panencephalitis (SSPE), and 'post-anoxic' myoclonus. Myoclonic jerks are seen in patients with absence seizures or partial seizures, in infantile spasms, and in the Lennox–Gastaut syndrome.

Progressive myoclonus epilepsy may be caused by a wide variety of conditions including Lafora body disease, neuronal ceroid liposfuscinosis, sialidosis, some forms of Gaucher's disease, dentatorubropallidoluyisan atrophy, neuroaxonal dystrophies, and the mitochondrial encephalopathies (Berkovic et al., 1986). Several inherited, geographically-defined variants have been reported. Both Unverricht–Lundborg or 'Baltic', and 'Mediterranean' myoclonus have a better prognosis than forms with a clear metabolic or pathologic abnormality (Koskiniemi et al., 1974; Genton et al., 1990). In infants, various 'benign' types of myoclonus can be distingushed from infantile spasms by their normal EEG (Fejerman, 1991).

Both patients with EPC and animal models of EPC show muscle jerks which are time-locked to EEG discharges; also present are increased somatosensory evoked potentials (SEPS) and sometimes movement or stimulus sensitivity (Kugelberg and Widen, 1954; Chauvel *et al.*, 1978). EPC can be mimicked by segmental spinal myoclonus. The latter, however, has no EEG correlate, and all the muscles involved are innervated by a single spinal segment (Shibasaki, 1991). EPC usually is associated with focal pathology and EEG discharges; patients may experience fluctuating spread of muscle involvement (Thomas *et al.*, 1977). Nystagmus as a sole manifestation has been reported (Furman *et al.*, 1990).

Atonic seizures may be caused by 'negative' myoclonus: a sudden brief cessation of EMG activity, preceded by an EEG spike (Shibasaki, 1991). Drop attacks can occur in partial seizures and in conditions such as brainstem ischemia, cataplexy or narcolepsy.

Myoclonic jerks and other movement disorders are common during sleep; polysomnography may be needed to distinguish them from seizures (Dyken and Rodnitsky, 1992). Several unusual movement disorders such as paroxysmal kinesiogenic choreoathetosis may be confused with myoclonus or seizures. An autosomal dominant dystonia, this disorder is induced by exercise or sensory stimulation; it is not associated with loss of consciousness or EEG changes, but may respond to AEDs (Stevens, 1966).

---

28 Clonic and tonic seizures are rare

Clonic (really a series of repeated myoclonic jerks) and tonic seizures are common in neonates (Principle 11). Tonic seizures are a prominent feature in the Lennox–Gastaut syndrome and may involve the neck and facial muscles alone or the arms and legs; brief apnea and a cry may occur (Blume, 1987). Patients with juvenile myoclonic epilepsy (Principle 23), or one of the other disorders in which myoclonus is a prominent feature (Principle 27), may be described as having clonic seizures, particularly if the jerks occur in clusters. Generalized clonic and tonic seizures rarely occur alone in older children and adults, but may precede GTCS (Theodore *et al.*, 1994b).

Isolated tonic seizures in older children and adults usually occur in patients with GTCS who have evidence of diffuse cerebral dysfunction rather than an unambiguous seizure focus (Spencer *et al.*, 1988). The attacks usually last about ten seconds, may have myoclonic components, begin and end abruptly or slowly, and are associated with a loss of consciousness (Gowers, 1885; Gastaut and Broughton, 1972). Head and eye deviation as well as facial contraction may be prominent features. The EEG usually shows bilateral flattening, low voltage fast activity, or a pattern similar to the tonic phase of GTCS. Autonomic features such as mydriasis, tachycardia, hypertension, glandular hypersecretion, and apnea may occur. The attacks are variable and clinically heterogeneous; they have shared features with GTCS that suggest that they are fragments of GTCS which are modified by drugs or other therapy. Patients with intracranial hypertension, cerebellar tumors, or multiple sclerosis may have paroxsymal episodes of increased tone which can be confused with seizures (Gastaut and Broughton, 1972; Matthews, 1976). These episodes may last one to two minutes, longer than true tonic seizures, and are not associated with epileptiform EEG activity. Tonic attacks in patients with multiple sclerosis may respond to carbamazepine. (Matthews, 1976).

Tonic head deviation may occur at the beginning of a complex partial seizure. There has been considerable disagreement whether the direction of deviation can be used to lateralize seizure onset (Ochs *et al.*, 1984; Wyllie *et al.*, 1986). Jayaker *et al.* (1992) have suggested that useful information can be obtained if the different actions of the two components of the sternocleidomastoid muscle are analyzed during videotape seizure analysis.

29 Patients with 'mixed seizures' have more than one seizure type

The term 'mixed seizures' properly refers to a patient with two or more types of classifiable epileptic seizures, such as a combination of generalized tonic–clonic seizures and absence seizures. The term is most often applied to children with Lennox–Gastaut syndrome; these children may indeed have several seizure types, including generalized tonic–clonic seizures, absence seizures, and atonic seizures. From the viewpoints of seizure classification and prognosis, it is important to obtain historical information on the various seizure types individually; only infrequently can this information not be obtained in the course of taking a detailed medical history. In the Lennox–Gastaut syndrome, the atonic spells may be much more resistant to therapy and restricting to the patient than the more severe, but more easily controlled generalized tonic–clonic attacks.

Unfortunately, the diagnosis 'mixed seizure disorder' often implies a paucity of information about the kinds of attacks the patient is having and reflects an inadequate medical history or inability to classify seizures, or both. The same is true for 'minor motor seizure', which is usually a euphemism for 'small seizure of unknown type, associated with movement'. The latter may refer, for example, to infantile spasms, atonic attacks, absence seizures with mild clonic components, or even simple partial seizures with clonic jerking. The diagnosis of minor motor seizures should be discarded in favor of the proper description of the seizure type.

6 Diagnosis: Status Epilepticus

> **30** Convulsive status epilepticus is a medical emergency

Status epilepticus, a condition in which seizures are so prolonged or so repeated that recovery does not occur between attacks, can be divided into generalized and partial status epilepticus. More useful clinically, however, is the division between convulsive and nonconvulsive status. Nonconvulsive status is described in Principle 31.

Convulsive (tonic–clonic) status epilepticus occurs when the patient has generalized tonic–clonic seizures so frequently that another seizure begins before the patient returns to normal consciousness from the postictal state; it is a medical emergency with a mortality rate of approximately 10%. It is essential that 'convulsive status [be] stopped as soon as possible...because the molecular events that lead to selective cell death are already operational during the first two to three convulsions' (Delgado-Escueta *et al.*, 1982). Tonic–clonic status is characterized, according to Gastaut (1983), by two types of seizures: primary generalized tonic–clonic attacks or, more frequently, secondarily generalized tonic–clonic seizures following a partial onset. The seizures themselves are typical generalized tonic–clonic seizures (Principle 20).

A predictable sequence of EEG changes in status has been observed (Treiman *et al.*, 1987; Treiman, 1993). Treiman has also described 'subtle' generalized status, in which movements are seen which are less vigorous than those in typical status; these include 'eyelid, facial, or jaw twitching, rhythmic nystagmoid eye jerks, or rhythmic subtle focal twitches of the trunk or extremities', all on a background of stupor or coma. This state can be caused by inadequate treatment of convulsive status and is deserving of immediate intervention (Treiman, 1993).

In patients with chronic epilepsy, one of the most common precipitating factors of status is failure of epileptic patients to take their antiepileptic drugs. Gumnit and Sell (1981) have described the most common causes of non-compliance leading to status epilepticus: (1) the patient may run out of medication and fail to renew the prescription, (2) the patient may take medication only sporadically, (3) the patient may lose the medication and not obtain another supply, (4) the patient, or the physician, may erroneously decide that anti-epileptic drugs are no longer needed, or (5) the patient may misunderstand the physician's instructions.

Tonic–clonic status is also more common in patients with known etiologies for their epilepsy (Janz, 1983). The search for the cause of the status epilepticus should therefore be vigorous, especially in older patients. Epileptic patients should be reevaluated if there is any doubt about the fundamental cause of the status epilepticus. In a series of 2,588 patients with epilepsy, Janz (1983) noted that only 1.6% of 1,885 patients with epilepsy of unknown cause had had a bout of status epilepticus, whereas 9% of patients with epilepsy of known cause had had tonic–clonic status; the most frequent causes of the epilepsy in the latter group were tumor or trauma. As noted by Treiman (1993), other important causes include CNS infection, cerebral infarction, drug abuse (see below) and human immunodeficiency virus (HIV) infection. Febrile seizures are a common cause of status in children under the age of three (Gross-Tsur and Shinnar, 1993).

In a study of 98 patients with generalized tonic–clonic status, Aminoff and Simon (1980) noted that, in their urban population, alcohol withdrawal was a major factor in 15 patients; a similar number had cerebrovascular disease as the cause of their status epilepticus. Other causes included intracranial infection, metabolic disorders, drug overdose, and cardiac arrest. In 15% of the patients, no specific cause could be found. Poor outcome correlated primarily with long-lasting status epilepticus. These investigators also noted that the status epilepticus was usually accompanied by hyperthermia and that the leukocyte count increased not only in the peripheral circulation but also in the CSF in 18% of the patients. The special consequences of status epilepticus in infants and children have been reviewed by Aicardi and Chevrie (1983).

Finally, it is important to note that status epilepticus with localizing features suggestive of partial seizures does not always indicate localized pathologic lesions. The phenomenon of partial or lateralized attacks has been associated in some patients with such diffuse cerebral insults as drug overdose or metabolic disturbance (Aminoff and Simon, 1980). Similar observations have been made in patients with hepatic encephalopathy; localized epileptic seizures do not necessarily mean localized pathologic change (Adams and Foley, 1953).

The therapy of generalized tonic–clonic status is discussed in Principles 82 and 83.

---

31 Nonconvulsive status epilepticus is a diagnostic problem

Although only convulsive (generalized tonic–clonic) status epilepticus is immediately life threatening, the various types of nonconvulsive status epilepticus, such as simple partial status (epilepsia partialis continua), complex partial status (psychomotor status) and petit mal status (spike-wave stupor), are often difficult diagnostic problems. Of the latter groups, petit mal status is the most varied in its nature and form (Porter and Penry, 1983).

Epilepsia partialis continua refers to persistent simple partial seizures, usually with motor manifestations but without a march, and usually remaining confined to the part of the body in which they originated. They may last for hours or days, and although consciousness is preserved, postictal weakness is commonly observed (Commission on Classification and Terminology of the International League Against Epilepsy, 1981) (see Figure 31.4).

Complex partial status is, unlike petit mal status, a *series* of complex partial seizures without intervening return to full responsiveness (Figure 31.1). The patient's condition cycles back and forth from a deep unresponsiveness during the actual partial seizures to mild-to-moderate alteration between attacks (Porter and Penry, 1983; Treiman and Delgado-Escueta, 1983). Complex partial status is rare, but occurs especially in patients who have severe, intractable complex partial seizures and who have, for some reason, discontinued their antiepileptic medication.

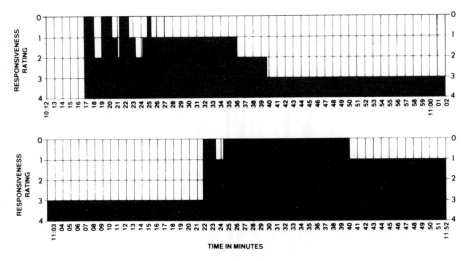

Figure 31.1 Responsiveness during complex partial status. The patient had a complex partial seizure at 10:17 a.m. and did not recover normal consciousness until several hours later. He had several attacks at the onset of status (10:17 a.m. to 10:25 a.m.), then appeared to be gradually recovering, but had another series of attacks beginning at 11:22 a.m. Recovery occurred gradually. The verbal responsiveness rating is as follows: 0 = no response; 1 = minimal response; 2 = comprehends, follows simple directions, identifies receptively, cannot answer verbally, anomia may be present; 3 = partial responsiveness, responds appropriately with one or two words and rote phrases, abnormal affect, some anomia; 4 = accurate and immediate response, normal affect, responds to others' comments, and initiates conversation, responds with more than one or two words (from Porter and Penry, 1983, with permission).

The importance of recognizing and treating complex partial status has been emphasized by Engel *et al.* (1978) who noted prolonged memory impairment in an 18-year-old girl with four episodes of complex partial status. Treiman and Delgado-Escueta (1983) also reported persistent short-term memory deficits in two patients with complex partial status. This entity is clearly not benign and requires immediate therapy (Krumholz *et al.*, 1986).

Petit mal status is known by a variety of names. The disorder is exceedingly heterogeneous, and the terminology has been reviewed (Porter and Penry, 1983). Only three criteria are applicable to this group of patients, but these are not diagnostic: (1) continuous (or nearly continuous) epileptiform EEG activity, usually generalized, is found; rarely, only generalized slowing will be noted, (2) behavioral change, usually associated with lethargy and decreased mental function, is present, and (3) there is absence of gross tonic–clonic activity.

The heterogeneity of patients with petit mal status is reflected in the wide variations in ictal EEGs. The classic, more or less continuous, 3-Hz spike-and-wave discharge has been described by many observers, and it probably correlates best with the typical absence seizure – such findings may form a subset of petit mal status and be termed 'absence status'. Other EEG findings include diverse spike-and-wave abnormalities, as well as continuous spikes or sharp waves. According to Porter and Penry (1983), 'it is safe to conclude from these data that virtually any generalized, continuous or nearly continuous abnormality could be a substrate for this syndrome'.

The state of altered consciousness may be extremely variable, both inter- and

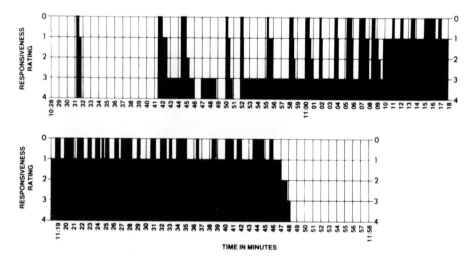

Figure 31.2 Responsiveness during petit mal status. The patient had a brief absence attack at 10:31 a.m., then a series of attacks beginning at 10:41 a.m., with intervening periods of normal responsiveness. She had severe impairment of responsiveness from 11:10 a.m. to 11:48 a.m., and then made a sudden recovery without postictal abnormality or complaint. The responsiveness rating is the same as in Figure 31.1 (from Porter and Penry, 1983, with permission).

PRINCIPLE 31

intra-individually (Figure 31.2). Some patients may be nearly normal, and, according to Andermann and Robb (1972), are 'only aware of a lack of efficiency', whereas others are barely responsive. Most patients are dull, confused, and lethargic; spontaneous activity is decreased. Often, such patients will demonstrate automatic behavior, and may even be able to eat, walk about, or follow simple commands (Porter and Penry, 1983). Mild myoclonia, especially of the eyelids, is also common.

The first attack of petit mal status may come at any age. In some patients, the first attack is the first manifestation of epilepsy (Figure 31.3).

Differentiation of petit mal status from complex partial status is important therapeutically, because antiepileptic drug therapy is different for each disorder. The most useful criterion is the medical history, which usually uncovers the underlying seizure type. Another useful criterion is the manner in which the attacks end. Petit mal status usually ends abruptly, without postictal abnormality, even after a prolonged episode (Figure 31.2), whereas complex partial status is associated with postictal depression, confusion, or malaise (Figure 31.1). Rarely, differentiation of petit mal status from two very unusual syndromes may

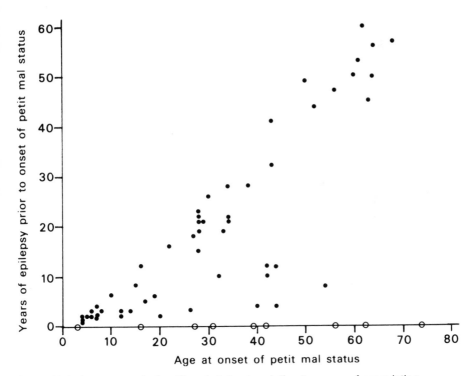

Figure 31.3 Age at onset of petit mal status in relation to years of preexisting epilepsy. Onset of petit mal status varied from 3 to 74 years of age in 53 patients with epilepsy for <1 to 63 years (filled circles). The first bout of petit mal status occurred at ages 3 to 73 in nine patients without a history of epilepsy (open circles) (from Porter and Penry, 1983, with permission).

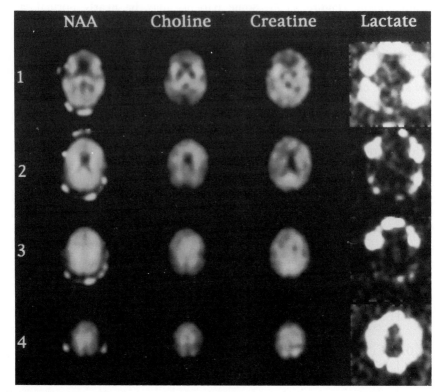

Figure 31.4 Magnetic resonance spectroscopy scan (slices 1–4) in a patient with epilepsia partialis continua, and twitching of the left hand and arm. There is no difference between the left and right hemisphere lactate signals, suggesting that a new metabolic equilibrium exists. MRS can be used to measure a number of metabolic parameters simultaneously.

be important; these are 'epilepsy with electrical status epilepticus during slow wave sleep', and the Landau–Kleffner syndrome (Cascino, 1993). Electro-encephalographic data may be decisive in some patients; if possible, an EEG during the ictal event is recommended.

7 Diagnosis: Nonepileptic Seizures and Febrile Seizures

> **32** Patients with refractory seizures sometimes do not have epilepsy

Almost fifteen years ago, Mattson (1980) reported that 22% of the patients referred to his clinic had not responded to previous antiepileptic drug therapy because they did not have epilepsy. In 1993, Gumnit noted that '15 to 20% of the patients admitted...had nonepileptic events, nearly all psychogenic'. These patients have nonepileptic attacks that resemble seizures of epileptic origin but which do not arise from abnormal neuronal discharge.

If the word 'seizure' is used in its broadest sense to include any paroxysmal attacks with apparent alteration of responsiveness, and/or motor, sensory, or autonomic dysfunction, then it is possible to construct a logical sequence of restrictive terms to describe these phenomena (Table 32.1). Epileptic seizures are most commonly encountered and are, by definition, caused by abnormal neuronal discharge. Other organic seizures involve other systems, such as the cardiovascular system. Metabolic disorders may also be associated with seizures. An overlap between epileptic and other organic seizures is apparent (Desai *et al.*, 1982). Nonorganic seizures are those in which no clear anatomic pathologic change can be correlated with the disorder.

In 84 patients with nonepileptic seizures studied by Mattson (1980), the most common attacks were associated with hysterical (psychogenic) causes (34 patients), drug toxicity (15 patients), and cerebral ischemia (10 patients). A surprising 75% of the patients improved after appropriate diagnosis and therapy.

Not all nonepileptic paroxysmal events can be considered in this volume. Excellent reviews by Pedley (1983) and by Pellock (1993) consider the differential diagnosis of gastroesophageal reflux of infants and young children, breath-holding spells, pallid infantile syndrome, sleep disorders (including the parasomnias – pavor nocturnus, somnambulism, enuresis and somniloquy), periodic nocturnal myoclonus, bruxism, headbanging, benign paroxysmal vertigo, transient global amnesia, transient ischemic attacks, migraine and other

Table 32.1 Common conditions associated with seizures or seizure-like phenomena

Organic conditions	Nonorganic conditions
Epileptic seizures	Psychogenic seizures*
Cardiovascular	Hysterical seizures*
Aortic stenosis	Conversion seizures*
Arrhythmias	Functional seizures*
Vasovagal	Pseudoseizures*
Orthostatic hypotension	
Transient cerebral ischemia	Other psychiatric disorders (such as
Movement disorders	schizophrenia)
Toxic or metabolic disorders	Malingering
Hypoglycemia	
Drug toxicity	
Sleep disorders	
Headache	

Modified and expanded from Mattson (1980), with permission.
*Terms marked with an asterisk are often used interchangeably.

nonepileptic paroxysmal disorders. Pseudoseizures, acute anxiety, and syncope present the most common differential problems in adults and will be considered in the following principles.

---

33 There is no absolute criterion for psychogenic seizures

The most frequently encountered of the nonepileptic seizures are psychogenic seizures, also called hysterical or pseudoseizures. The following is exemplary:

A twelve-year-old girl was healthy until she experienced her first seizure at an educational overnight camp. The patient was described as being unresponsive, with her arms and legs shaking. The episode lasted 20 minutes, but was not associated with incontinence, tongue biting, or postictal abnormality. She had no memory for the attack. An EEG was reported as 'consistent with psychomotor seizures', and phenytoin was prescribed. During phenytoin therapy, the patient had several witnessed attacks, which began with an interruption of movement and were followed by falling forward or backward, without evident trauma; jerking of all four extremities might then last from a few seconds to a minute. She developed Stevens–Johnson syndrome and was hospitalized in an intensive care unit. Phenobarbital was started, but the seizures persisted. Carbamazepine and then primidone were added to the regimen, but the attacks continued. The patient was referred for intensive inpatient evaluation of her seizures.

The results of the neurologic examination and the EEG were normal. Two attacks were recorded; in each attack, the patient gradually fell forward and was unresponsive. She returned quickly to normal consciousness following the attacks, which lasted 10 to 20 seconds. No changes were observed in the EEG during the attacks.

The patient's medications were gradually tapered. She stated spontaneously that she could control all her attacks, and she was discharged, seizure-free, on no medication. Follow-up one year later revealed no recurrence of seizures.

Psychogenic seizures are surprisingly common. They are also often difficult to diagnose accurately, and are often mistakenly treated with antiepileptic drugs. Errors of diagnosis and, therefore, of treatment are compounded by the attending physician's erroneous desire to make a hasty diagnosis on the basis of second-hand evidence or even after witnessing an attack. Sometimes it is simply not possible, by observation, to determine the etiology of a seizure, and a considered, rational opinion can be offered only after all data have been collected. According to Desai et al. (1982), the most useful data are provided by simultaneous video and EEG recording of the attacks, recording of the ictal and postictal EEG, and observation of the relationship between antiepileptic medication and seizure frequency (Table 33.1). These criteria are best applied in a setting of intensive monitoring, which may be the only definitive method of establishing the diagnosis (Desai et al., 1982). A comprehensive volume considers all aspects of these attacks (Rowan and Gates, 1993).

Recorded attacks

The heterogeneity of psychogenic seizures is limited only by the machinations of the human mind. Although epileptic patients with frontal lesions may have bizarre automatisms (Williamson et al., 1985; Williamson, 1993), epileptic seizures usually have a comparatively limited and stereotyped clinical expression. If the suspected attack is recorded and compared with epileptic seizures of known etiology, using the international classification of epileptic seizures, a diagnosis by exclusion is often possible. This assumption has three axioms: (1) some patients will have psychogenic attacks that do not resemble either generalized tonic–clonic or complex partial seizures, (2) a certain small but finite group of epileptic seizures will be characterized by unusual events that make classification difficult, and (3) the more experienced the physician in the observation of all types of seizures, the more likely the seizure classification will be correct (Desai et al., 1982).

Ictal and postictal EEG

The EEG is almost always abnormal during an epileptic seizure, especially if consciousness is altered. This observation is helpful in confirming the diagnosis

Table 33.1 Major criteria useful for diagnosing either epileptic or psychogenic seizures

| Characteristics | Epileptic seizures | | Nonepileptic seizures |
	Generalized tonic–clonic seizures	Complex partial seizures	Psychogenic seizures
Comparison of questionable seizure with known seizure types*	Relatively little variation in events	Wide range of events, but most common are well described	Extremely wide range of events with bizarre and unusual behavior
EEG during seizure	Abnormal and changed from preictal	Almost always abnormal and changed from preictal	Usually normal and unchanged from preictal
EEG immediately after seizure	Almost always abnormal and changed from preictal	Frequently abnormal and changed from preictal	Usually normal and unchanged from preictal
Relation of attacks to medication regimen	Prominent, especially in severely affected patients	Usually related	Usually unrelated

*As described in the international classification of epileptic seizures (Gastaut, 1970).
From Desai et al. (1982).

of epilepsy even though many different paroxysmal abnormalities can be observed, especially in partial seizures. Two problems arise in the effective utilization of this criterion. First, in a small percentage of patients with epileptic seizures, the ictal EEG will not show abnormalities. Second, the ictal EEG is often obscured by movement and muscle artifact, regardless of the etiology of the attack. A good quality recording of the ictal EEG, however, makes a valuable contribution to the diagnosis. The EEG is almost always abnormal after a generalized tonic–clonic seizure and is frequently abnormal after a complex partial seizure. The postictal EEG has one chief advantage over the ictal EEG: it is less often obscured by artifact, and interpretation of the recording may be easier.

Medication and seizure frequency

As Desai et al. (1982) have stated, properly treated epileptic patients show a strong tendency to have fewer seizures when plasma levels of antiepileptic drugs are adequate. This relationship between medications and seizure regulation can be useful in the assessment of suspected psychogenic seizures. The best procedure is to withdraw medications gradually while the patient is in the hospital and observe for increases in seizure frequency. The use of intensive monitoring to record the increased seizure frequency during medication withdrawal enhances the likelihood of a correct diagnosis.

Numerous other, less important, criteria have been utilized in an attempt to discern which seizures are psychogenic (Table 33.2) and which are epileptic (Table 33.3).

Psychogenic seizures are more difficult to diagnose when they look like complex partial seizures than when they look like generalized tonic–clonic seizures. When the latter is the case, data are available to assist in the bedside diagnosis. Gates *et al.* (1985) studied spontaneous psychogenic seizures which resembled generalized tonic–clonic seizures and compared these attacks to epileptic

Table 33.2 Minor criteria primarily used for diagnosing suspected psychogenic seizures

	Epileptic seizures		Nonepileptic seizures
Characteristics	Generalized tonic–clonic seizures	Complex partial seizures	Psychogenic seizures
Onset	Usually paroxysmal, but may be preceded by seizure of different type	Usually paroxysmal, but may be preceded by aura of only a few seconds	Often gradual; prolonged nonspecific warning period may occur
Primary or secondary gain	Rare; a few patients use seizures for secondary gain	Unusual, but a few patients use seizures for secondary gain	Common
Postictal confusion, lethargy, sleepiness	Prominent	Almost always present and often prominent but may be mild	Often conspicuously absent; patient may be normal immediately after attack
Postictal subjective complaints	Prominent if aroused	Usually prominent; patient rarely feels well	May be smiling or laughing after seizure
Suggestibility	None	Rare	Occasionally
Recollection of events during attack	None	Usually scant and most often none	Sometimes detailed
Violent behavior	None	Rare; virtually always in response to restraint and not highly directed	Rare, though may be highly directed

From Desai *et al.* (1982).

PRINCIPLE 33

Table 33.3 Minor criteria primarily useful for diagnosing suspected epileptic seizures

	Epileptic seizures		Nonepileptic seizures
Characteristics	Generalized tonic–clonic seizures	Complex partial seizures	Psychogenic seizures
Age	Any, past infancy	Any, usually >3 years	Usually older child or adult
Gross tonic–clonic motor phenomena	Always	Rare; seen only in secondarily generalized attacks	None, but resemblance is related to sophistication of mimicry
Tongue biting	Frequent	Rare	Rare
Urinary incontinence	Frequent	Unusual, but not rare	Rare
Abnormal neurologic signs during seizure	May be present	May be present	None
Nocturnal occurrence	Common	May occur	Rare
Injuries sustained as a result of event	Common	Common	Rare, but occasionally occur
Stereotypy of attacks	Relatively little variation	Attacks may or may not be varied, but usually have some consistent patterns	Attacks may or may not be varied; patterns may occasionally be widely divergent

From Desai *et al.* (1982).

generalized tonic–clonic seizures. In comparison to epileptic attacks, the psychogenic seizures were (1) more likely in women, (2) often longer or shorter than epileptic generalized tonic–clonic seizures, (3) had out-of-phase upper and lower extremity movements, (4) tended to thrust the pelvis forward, and (5) had body rigidity which was less pronounced.

Unfortunately, the positive diagnosis of psychogenic seizures is rarely possible, and no single criterion should be singled out as diagnostic. Attempts to formulate positive criteria for psychogenic seizures by using either personality traits (Vanderzant *et al.*, 1986) or psychometric testing (Henrichs *et al.*, 1988) have not been successful. The diagnosis remains one of exclusion of other conditions. Also, the separation of hysteria from malingering is often impossible.

It is possible to utilize serum prolactin levels to exclude some patients with epilepsy who are suspected of having psychogenic seizures (Sperling *et al.*, 1986).

PRINCIPLE 33

Certain epileptic seizures cause hyperprolactinemia. Generalized tonic–clonic and complex partial seizures of temporal lobe origin yield the most consistent rises. Extratemporal seizures – especially simple partial seizures not involving temporal structures – may not increase prolactin levels. Mild elevations may be seen in patients with pseudoseizures (Laxer *et al.*, 1985), and the criteria for a 'significant' prolactin rise from baseline remains a topic of discussion. Postictal prolactin levels peak at 15 minutes (Sperling *et al.*, 1986); later collection of samples may not be useful. In summary, although a prominent prolactin rise strongly suggests epilepsy and although some centers use such a rise to document convulsive epileptic seizures (King *et al.*, 1993), the lack of such an increase is not diagnostic of psychogenic seizures (Yerby *et al.*, 1987). Furthermore, many patients with psychogenic seizures will also have epileptic attacks.

Psychogenic seizures are often associated with psychiatric disturbances other than 'hysteria' or 'somatoform disorder' (Gates and Erdahl, 1993) In fact, depression and schizophrenia are common underlying psychiatric conditions which promote the symptoms of hysteria. Physicians confronted with a patient with apparent psychogenic seizures, therefore, should apply the above criteria and should not be dissuaded by a seemingly inconsistent overall psychiatric diagnosis. As noted above, intensive video and EEG monitoring can be very helpful (Meierkord *et al.*, 1991; Porter and Sato, 1993). The disorder may occur in the elderly (Fakhoury *et al.*, 1993) and can even occur in early childhood; Duchowney *et al.* (1988) used intensive monitoring to identify 24 pseudoseizure patients under the age of ten.

Hyperventilation frequently accompanies psychogenic seizures and is accompanied by tetany as well as dizziness, blurred vision, paresthesias, shortness of breath, and other symptoms (Riley and Roy, 1982; Pedley, 1983). One type of psychogenic seizures is especially difficult to discern from atonic seizures. Patients, in this group, usually young women, fall without convulsive movements. They may be incontinent of urine, especially if they discover that it will worry their doctors (Walton, 1985; Meierkord *et al.*, 1991).

Finally, patients with psychogenic seizures, even though they may not have epilepsy, are ill and require psychiatric evaluation and care. One approach to therapy is introduction of the concept that the patient can control the attacks. This concept should be introduced slowly, allowing a graceful exit from the psychogenic seizures. Occasionally, the attacks will stop abruptly when the patient is confronted directly; if this technique fails, however, rapport may be lost that might have allowed cessation of the attacks. Therapy of psychogenic seizures is considered in detail by Riley and Roy (1982) and by Gumnit (1993a), who emphasizes the need to tailor the treatment to the individual patient.

---

34 Acute anxiety attacks are sometimes mistaken for epileptic seizures

---

Increasing recognition of the symptoms of anxiety, coupled with increased incidence of the disorder, has heightened awareness of the acute anxiety attack or panic attack. The attack itself may take many forms, but the common feature is an overwhelming sense of fear or panic. The fear may be 'free floating' or directed, and although often related to interpersonal encounters, attacks may also occur when the patient is completely alone. Patients are especially vulnerable 'when unaccompanied in the street, in crowds, buses, shops, and particularly when inactive or compelled to wait, as in cinemas or queues' (Harper and Roth, 1962). Recently, some investigators have noted the coexistence of panic disorder with epilepsy (Spitz, 1991; Stagno, 1993).

Psychophysiologic accompaniments of the attacks include intense sweating, 'spaced-out' or 'detached' feelings, sensations of unreality, palpitations, tachycardia, chest tightness, nausea, vomiting, diarrhea, and dyspnea. Exhaustion may follow an attack. The following is a typical case report:

A 36-year-old woman, an important and fast-rising executive, noticed the onset of 'being detached from the environment', a feeling which came on suddenly while drinking with her friends. The onset was paroxysmal and disappeared when she was able to go the bathroom. She had a similar episode a few weeks later and fainted, with loss of consciousness for approximately 20 seconds. She had no further alterations of consciousness but began having attacks' of panic, with associated feelings of coldness, perspiration, and 'a feeling of detachment', lasting from half a minute up to many hours, and occurring both at home and at work. A neurologist prescribed phenytoin, which caused her to feel worse, followed by primidone, which made her vomit. She took no medication for 2 months.

The results of the neurologic examination were normal, but the EEG showed left posterior temporal irregular slowing. A diagnosis of acute anxiety attacks was made, and the patient was given diazepam (4 mg/day) as needed for the attacks. She responded dramatically, with striking relief of the severity and frequency of her attacks. A later trial of antidepressant medication was not tolerated. Four years later, she continued to use the diazepam, though usually only once every few months.

The diagnosis of acute anxiety attacks usually rests on three factors. First, the duration of some of the attacks is quite prolonged, up to 15 to 30 minutes or more – much longer than most epileptic seizures. Second, consciousness is usually not altered during the attack; even though the patient may feel strange, appropriate interaction with the environment is still possible. The patient can very often recite in detail the events and his or her own actions during the attack (unless fainting occurs, as in the patient described above). Hyperventilation may be a prominent feature. Third, the EEG usually does not show epileptiform abnormalities, and is most often completely normal.

Sheehan (1982) was among the first to document the effectiveness of antidepressants for patients with severe, repetitive episodes of acute anxiety. Most patients respond to either tricyclic antidepressants, monoamine oxidase inhibitors or benzodiazepines such as alprazolam (Modigh, 1987). Benzodiazepine therapy is controversial, although diazepam is often effective initially, especially in milder cases. The therapy should be personalized, as noted by Matuzas and Jack (1991), who state that 'an approach characterized by flexibility and willingness to negotiate treatment plans with individual patients provides the greatest possibility of success'.

---

35 Prolonged fugue states are rarely epileptic if highly organized behavior occurs

Every neurologist is occasionally called upon to consider the possibility of epilepsy in patients who have prolonged attacks (i.e., hours or days) of altered responsiveness to their environment. In most such cases, the medical causes have already been adequately addressed, and the remaining differential diagnosis is between epilepsy and psychiatric disease. More specifically, it is usually between nonconvulsive status epilepticus (Principle 31) and a dissociative disorder. Several kinds of dissociative disorders can be confused with epilepsy. The following descriptions are taken largely from the draft version of *Diagnostic and Statistical Manual of Mental Disorders* – DSM-IV (American Psychiatric Association, 1993).

Dissociative amnesia is characterized by one or more episodes of inability to recall important personal information, usually of a traumatic or stressful nature; the disturbance is much more than ordinary forgetfulness. Typically, the patient fails to recall all events occurring during a circumscribed period of time.

The patient with a *dissociative fugue* makes a sudden, unexpected trip away from home or work, may assume a new identity, and may be confused and disoriented with inability to recall the past. Typically, the patient denies any recollection of the events during the fugue.

The patient with *multiple personality disorder* has at least two personalities or personality states that alternately become dominant. Epilepsy is sometimes considered in such patients when the change from one personality to the other is sudden, resembling the paroxysmal onset of a seizure. Misdiagnosis is common; in one study using intensive monitoring, six patients previously diagnosed as having multiple personality disorder and epilepsy were shown to have only psychogenic seizures (Devinsky *et al.*, 1989b).

Finally, the patient with *depersonalization disorder* has a feeling that the usual sense of one's own reality is temporarily lost or changed; a feeling of detachment or unreality pervades the patient's perceptions of his surroundings (Principle 19).

The key to the diagnosis can usually be found in a historical analysis of the complexity of the tasks performed during the event. If the patient can barely carry out the tasks of daily living, such as eating and drinking, a continuous seizure state must be considered and evaluated intensively. If, however, the patient disappears from home for two days, then calls home from a distant city and says that he doesn't know what happened or how he got there, then a psychiatric disorder is most likely. A psychiatric diagnosis is especially likely if a number of complicated transactions can be documented during the event, (e.g., changing airplanes, making purchases, arranging accommodations). The more intricate and complicated the overall performance, the less likely the behavior is to be epileptic. This fundamental observation also applies to complicated tasks performed during aggressive behavior in which epilepsy is considered in the differential diagnosis (Principle 37). The differentiation of anxiety attacks from transient global amnesia and from the amnesia which follows a complex partial seizure (Andermann, 1993) is important.

---

36 Clonic jerking or tonic extension may accompany syncopal episodes

---

The neurologist is frequently confronted with a patient who has paroxysmal episodes of alteration of consciousness, with loss of postural tone and clonic jerking and/or tonic extension. In many such patients, the correct diagnosis is not epilepsy but syncope. The following case illustrates the problem:

A 17-year-old girl was well until the age of 2 years, when she fell and was unresponsive for 1 minute; thereafter, she was somewhat 'groggy'. A second, similar episode occurred 4 days later, and although the neurologic examination and EEG showed no abnormalities, she was started on phenobarbital, which she took to the age of 6 years. She had only one further episode, when she was 4 years old.

At 10 years of age, she had loss of consciousness and a few jerking movements at the time of a venipuncture. She then began having attacks several times a year, characterized by loss of consciousness, loss of postural tone, tonic flexion of the arms, and extension of the legs. The attacks lasted 30 to 60 seconds and were followed by postictal confusion and headache. They were preceded by dimming of central vision and a feeling of dizziness. She was advised to seek psychiatric care. By the age of 18 years, she was having one or two attacks a month, and was hospitalized for intensive monitoring because of a sudden increase in attacks to 15 a month. A typical episode was precipitated by venipuncture; dramatic EKG evidence of sinus bradycardia and sinus arrest was documented during the attack.

Table 36.1 Causes of cardiogenic syncope

I.   Drop in cardiac output

     Hypovolemia
         Blood loss
         Excessive diuretics
         Fluid loss

     Decreased venous tone
         Nitrates
         Calcium channel blockers
         Sympathetic blockade

     Sudden obstruction to blood flow
         Atrial myxoma
         Pulmonary embolism

     Disease where ability to increase cardiac output is limited
         Aortic stenosis
         Idiopathic hypertrophic subaortic stenosis
         Pulmonary hypertension

     Disease affecting local cerebral blood flow
         Carotid artery embolism or thrombosis
         Dissection of aorta

     Disease interfering with cardiac filling
         Pericardial tamponade

II.   Reflex syncope (inappropriate drop in systemic vascular resistance and/or heart rate)

     Vasodepressor (vasovagal) syncope

     Carotid sinus syncope

     Other reflex triggers (glossopharyngeal, post-micturition, post-tussive, ocular, splanchnic, cerebral, esophageal)

     Inappropriate vasodepressor reflexes
         Aortic stenosis

III.   Sudden drop in systemic vascular resistance

     Drugs
         Vasodilators
         Antihypertensives
         Antisympathetic drugs

     Autonomic nervous system dysfunction
         Primary
         Secondary (diabetes, amyloidosis)

IV.   Arrhythmias

     Bradyarrhythmias (sick sinus syndrome)

     Heart block

     Tachyarrhythmias
         Atrial (fibrillation, flutter, Wolf–Parkinson–White)
         Ventricular (tachycardia, fibrillation)

From Dohrmann and Cheitlin (1986), with permission.

PRINCIPLE 36

Syncope usually refers to cardiogenic syncope, and is related to a sudden drop in cerebral blood flow (Dohrmann and Cheitlin, 1986). The various syncopal syndromes have been subdivided into three major and two minor categories by Riley (1982), and into four categories by Dohrmann and Cheitlin (1986). Table 36.1 lists the surprisingly numerous causes of this disorder. The relationship to epilepsy has been further reviewed by Niedermeyer (1993b).

The differential diagnosis of epilepsy and syncope is highly dependent on an adequate medical history. The setting of the attacks may be an important clue to their etiology. Some patients, such as the one just described, have stereotyped causes of their attacks; common precipitating factors include sight of blood, venipuncture, minor trauma, or being in a warm crowded place (Pellock, 1993). Many of the same psychologically stressful environments associated with acute anxiety attacks (Principle 34) are implicated in syncope as well, and psychogenic attacks, including hyperventilation, must also be considered. Syncope can be precipitated in some patients by nonanxiety-related events, such as micturition and coughing. Patients with syncope often have a prolonged prodrome; the aura in epileptic attacks is usually only a few seconds. Although a few clonic jerks are common in syncope, and tonic extension also occurs (Aminoff *et al.*, 1988), the classic sequence of the generalized tonic–clonic epileptic seizure is rare. The diagnosis can be difficult to establish if the attacks occur while sitting or lying down (Andermann, 1993) or if the attacks are infrequent (Hoefnagels *et al.*, 1992). If the spells are frequent or precipitable, monitoring and simultaneous recording of the EEG and electrocardiogram (EKG) is usually definitive. The use of the ambulatory EEG monitor is beneficial when one lead is used to record the EKG (Lai and Ziegler, 1981).

In the 17-year-old girl described above, the vasovagal syncope was unresponsive to cardiac pacing or atropine, demonstrating that bradycardia was not the sole cause of the hypotension. She responded to the use of elastic stockings and leg exercises to minimize the peripheral pooling, which was apparently the result of centrally induced vasodepression (Goldstein *et al.*, 1982).

---

37 Aggression and violence are extremely uncommon during epileptic seizures

Most epileptiologists agree that violence (the *act* of attempting to inflict damage) during or after an epileptic seizure occurs almost exclusively in a setting of direct provocation and is more likely to occur in the postictal period. Aggression (the *intent* to inflict harm) is even rarer (Stagno, 1993).

In an international workshop involving 16 epilepsy centers, 19 epileptic seizures with possible violent behavior were identified from an estimated 5,400 recorded seizures. Eighteen experts from these centers evaluated the 19 attacks by repeated viewing of the videotaped seizures. Three attacks were thought to show actual or threatened violence to persons (Delgado-Escueta *et al.*, 1981b). The most severe, violent act was an attempt to scratch another person's face, an act that was typical of the patient's seizures. Depth electrode stimulation of the left hippocampus caused a typical violent seizure (Saint-Hilare *et al.*, 1980). Even this patient could be restrained if held from behind.

The rarity of violence as an ictal event in epileptic patients is supported by the incidence of 0.00019 for unprovoked violence in the highly selected patient population from these referral centers. Such centers specialize in the most difficult and refractory patients.

Although it is admittedly difficult to prove the nonexistence of ictal violence in epilepsy, conclusions drawn from the above findings can be applied to the vast majority of patients with epilepsy: (1) automatic behavior during seizures is usually brief, fragmentary, and nondirected; most epileptic automatisms are less effective and less directed than normal behavior in the same setting; (2) the more complex and more prolonged the activity, the less likely it is to be epileptic. Complicated acts of violence, therefore, are highly unlikely to be epileptic in origin. With regard to interictal violence, one study suggests that underlying psychopathology and mental retardation are more important factors than seizure variables (Mendez *et al.*, 1993).

From the above, one can conclude that the use of epilepsy as a defense against accusations of violent and aggressive crime is virtually always unwarranted. In a comprehensive review of this issue by Treiman (1986), criteria were suggested for determining whether or not an act of violence was the result of an epileptic seizure. These are: (1) establishment of the diagnosis of epilepsy by a neurologist with special competence in epilepsy, (2) documentation of automatisms and aggression by history and video/EEG recording, and (3) agreement by the neurologist not only that the aggressive act is characteristic of patient's habitual seizures but that the specific violent act in question was part of a seizure.

38 Febrile seizures are common and usually benign

Febrile seizures are usually generalized tonic–clonic seizures, but can be classified on the basis of their clinical pattern. 'Simple' febrile seizures last less than 15 minutes, have no focal features or postictal neurologic deficit, and do not occur in clusters (Nelson and Ellenberg, 1981; Verity and Golding, 1991). 'Complex' febrile seizures are associated with one or more of these complicating features.

Children experiencing their first seizure at the time of fever need to be evaluated for infection or other possible etiologies. However, 'febrile seizures' are very common, occurring in 3–4% of children (Hirtz, 1989). About one-third have repeated febrile seizures, usually within two years. The risk of recurrence may be higher if (1) the patient has a family history of seizures, (2) the first attack occurred at less than 18 months, and (3) a short duration fever or relatively low temperature occurred before the seizure (Berg *et al.*, 1992; Offringa *et al.*, 1992).

The relation between febrile seizures and the development of repeated afebrile seizures (epilepsy) is unclear. Surgical series of patients with uncontrolled epilepsy often report a high incidence of remote febrile seizures; the attacks were often prolonged or complex. Mesial temporal sclerosis is the most common pathological finding; tumors are rare and the surgical outcome is good (Abou-Khalil *et al.*, 1993). Patients with drug-resistant partial seizures and MRI evidence of hippocampal volume loss may be more likely to have a history of febrile seizures (Kuks *et al.*, 1993). However, these studies all suffer from an obvious ascertainment bias and cannot be used to predict outcome for the usual child presenting with febrile seizures. Formal epidemiological studies, for example, suggest that less than 3% of children with febrile seizures will develop nonfebrile seizures by the age of 10 (Nelson and Ellenberg, 1981; Verity and Golding, 1991); the risk of recurrent febrile seizures is considerably greater (Figure 38.1). Risk factors for development of epilepsy may include febrile seizures lasting more

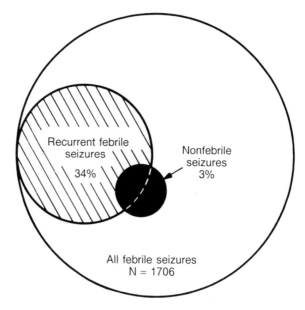

Figure 38.1 In a study of 1706 children with febrile seizures followed to the age of 7 years (*outer circle*), one-third had recurrent febrile seizures (*hatched circle*). Children with subsequent nonfebrile seizures (epilepsy) came almost equally from among those who did, and those who did not, have at least one recurrence of their febrile seizures (from Nelson and Ellenberg, 1981, with permission).

than 20 minutes, focal features, multiple episodes within 24 hours, associated neurologic impairment, and family history of seizures (Nelson and Ellenberg, 1976; Annegers *et al.*, 1987; Verity *et al.*, 1993). Patients with simple febrile seizures are much less likely to develop afebrile seizures by the age of 10 than those with complex febrile seizures (Nelson and Ellenberg, 1981; Verity and Golding, 1991).

8 Therapy: General Considerations

---

39 Be certain that the patient has epilepsy before prescribing antiepileptic drugs

---

Antiepileptic drugs are primarily useful for the treatment of recurrent abnormal neuronal discharges – epilepsy. Other conditions, such as bipolar depression, myotonia, and trigeminal neuralgia, may also be treated with certain antiepileptic drugs; Klawans (1979) has summarized several such uses; Bowden *et al.* (1994) recently documented the effectiveness of divalproex in mania. Unfortunately, since many patients with well-documented epilepsy continue to have seizures, physicians become inured to the many patients who, though their seizures are properly diagnosed and properly treated, simply do not get better. True though this may be for many patients with intractable seizures, the resulting attitude of hopelessness causes a failure to recognize that some patients who fail to respond to treatment have either the wrong diagnosis or the wrong therapy.

Epilepsy should virtually always be a positive diagnosis; when the diagnosis is uncertain, a therapeutic trial of antiepileptic drugs is rarely successful. When psychogenic seizures are incorrectly diagnosed as epilepsy, for example, administration of antiepileptic drugs may result in a temporary placebo effect, temporary worsening of the condition, or intolerance to the medication. Eventually, confusion reigns as more drugs at higher doses are tried. The chief pitfalls in the diagnosis of epilepsy include not only psychogenic seizures (Principle 33) but also acute anxiety attacks (Principle 34), dissociative states (Principle 35), and syncope (Principle 36).

Numerous studies have shown that a single drug controls seizures in many patients and that 'polytherapy' is often unnecessary. Refractory epilepsy, however, will often be better controlled with more than one drug (Porter *et al.*, 1980, Lorenzo *et al.*, 1988). The concept of monotherapy is reviewed in detail in Principle 41.

One area of particular concern to pediatricians is the proper diagnosis of 'abdominal epilepsy'. The epigastric aura (with or without a 'rising sensation') is the most common premonitory symptom in complex partial seizures, and abdominal symptoms also occur in children with seizures. Vomiting and abdominal pain may occur in association with altered responsiveness, other signs of epilepsy, and abnormal EEG findings. The onset of the attacks is usually paroxysmal, and postictal sleepiness is the rule. Although the diagnosis is frequently considered, especially in children who have recurrent episodes of abdominal pain and vomiting, 'only a small proportion of these children have abdominal epilepsy' (Menkes, 1985), even if a gastrointestinal evaluation is unrevealing. The diagnosis should not be made on the basis of the abdominal symptoms alone, but on the positive criteria noted above. Childhood migraine should especially be considered in the differential diagnosis.

---

40 The seizure diagnosis determines the appropriate therapy

The kinds of seizures that a patient has determine the correct medication or other therapy. This highly empirical approach still predominates in spite of continuing efforts to establish more basic and more rational diagnostic methods. The likelihood that basic neuroscience will contribute to the precise diagnosis of epilepsy still seems many years away. We do know, however, that the antiepileptic drugs now available are often quite specific for various types of epileptic seizures and that proper seizure classification (Principle 13) is crucial to appropriate therapy.

The clinical evidence for specificity of antiepileptic drugs against various seizure types is impressive. Consider the following information:

1. Some drugs, such as phenytoin or carbamazepine, are virtually ineffective against absence seizures or myoclonic seizures, but control most partial seizures and generalized tonic–clonic seizures.
2. Some drugs, such as ethosuximide or trimethadione, have no effect against partial seizures, generalized tonic–clonic seizures, or myoclonic seizures, but are useful in treating absence seizures.
3. Valproate is effective against both absence seizures and myoclonic seizures as well as primarily generalized tonic–clonic seizures.
4. Corticotropin (ACTH) may stop infantile spasms, but has little effect on other seizure types.

Although the basic mechanism of each of the seizure types is presumably related to the different response to various drugs, we still have incomplete information on these seizure mechanisms and about how antiepileptic drugs act to prevent their occurrence. Experimental data suggest that the variability of the various seizure types and their differential response to medication is complex.

As we are likely to continue with empirical rather than rational therapy for a considerable time to come, the refinement of empirical approaches has a legitimate role for both practitioners and clinical investigators.

---

41 Monotherapy is like motherhood – it's not for everyone

Much has been written in the past few years regarding the merits of monotherapy, which has been canonized as the only reasonable approach to antiepileptic drug therapy, especially as compared to the evils of multiple drug regimens, or 'polytherapy'. The latter, which merely means the use of more than one drug at a time in a single patient, has been declared unnecessary and inappropriate in a somewhat mindless way, without adequate and reasoned consideration that multiple drugs may, in fact, be useful in some patients. Monotherapy, therefore, tends to be treatment by slogan rather than by reason. The following statements (modified from Porter, 1989) consider the arguments both for and against monotherapy.

The best state of health is the medication-free state

While this statement is, on its own, self-evident, it points out that any therapy – including monotherapy – is inferior to a drug-free state when such a state is possible. Some patients with epilepsy prefer to risk an occasional seizure than risk toxicity from drug therapy. Others benefit so little from therapy that they may be better off without medication. Such patients are uncommon, but clearly monotherapy is second-best to the absence of therapy when none is needed or indicated. Finally, and perhaps most important, some patients who once required medical therapy may no longer need it and deserve a trial of drug withdrawal.

The advantages of limiting the total antiepileptic drug intake (either in number or in quantity) are well documented

When a single drug is taken to excess, both physician and patient become aware of the consequences; dose-related adverse effects are obvious, and the patient becomes ill. Less obvious is the advantage of taking fewer total numbers of medications. It is agreed by most, however, that the administration of fewer antiepileptic drugs has certain inherent advantages:

1. Adverse drug–drug interactions are much less likely; they obviously do not even occur with monotherapy.
2. Side effects in general may be fewer; a good example is the study by Kuzniecky *et al.* (1992) who evaluated post-surgery patients. This complex issue is further discussed in Principle 42.
3. Compliance by the patient may be better. However, compliance problems may also relate to inadequate attention by the physician to this issue.
4. Cost may be lower. It may also be higher if more expensive drugs are chosen.
5. Seizure control is better in some patients. But improvement in seizure control may not relate to a fundamental alteration in the propensity to have seizures. It may, rather, relate to increased compliance because of few adverse side effects.

A multi-drug regimen may occasionally be superior to monotherapy

In certain patients, almost always with severe, difficult-to-control epilepsy, multiple drugs appear to be more effective than single medications. Some data are specifically available on this issue from the multicenter Veterans Administration study of partial and generalized tonic–clonic seizures (Mattson *et al.*, 1985). Of 522 patients who were entered into this controlled trial, 82 were considered failures on monotherapy and were placed on a two-drug regimen. Of these, almost 40% were judged to be improved by such a regimen and nine patients (11%) became seizure-free. Furthermore, in an intensive study of 12 inpatients with intractable partial seizures, Lorenzo *et al.*, (1988) observed a significant improvement – without increased toxicity – using carbamazepine and phenytoin together as compared to each drug used alone; Finally, Dean *et al.* (1988), in a retrospective study, observed improvement using a combination of carbamazepine and valproate. Although only a minority of patients may respond, the physician should not automatically reject a multi-drug regimen as having no potential benefit for the patient.

A nonsedative regimen may be more important than monotherapy

In the past decade an increasing number of studies have suggested that certain antiepileptic drugs, notably those with sedative–hypnotic effects, may cause drowsiness and cognitive dysfunction in many patients with epilepsy. If one accepts that barbiturates and benzodiazepines are, with certain limited exceptions, 'second-line' antiepileptic drugs because of their sedating properties, then

PRINCIPLE 41

the physician should emphasize the use of the four older nonsedative antiepileptic drugs (phenytoin, carbamazepine, valproic acid, ethosuximide) or one of the newer drugs such as felbamate, gabapentin, lamotrigine, or vigabatrin.

Logically, one should begin therapy with one of these drugs as monotherapy. When a multi-drug regimen is indicated, combinations of nonsedative medications are preferable to combinations including barbiturates or benzodiazepines. Whether monotherapy with barbiturates or benzodiazepines is worth the effort before embarking on a multi-drug regimen has not been adequately investigated by clinical trials; only scant data are available to support a regimen of monotherapy with sedative-hypnotic antiepileptic drugs except for (1) certain specific seizure types such as the myoclonias which may respond to chronic benzodiazepine therapy and (2) patients who are intolerant of the usual first-line drugs.

In summary, when treatment is needed for epileptic seizures, all patients should first be tried on a single medication. This medication should, before being abandoned as ineffective, be 'pushed' gently to the point of dose-related side effects. Should the first medication fail, a second trial of a single agent should probably be attempted before considering a multi-drug regimen. A few patients, however, will have their epilepsy optimally controlled on multiple drugs.

---

42 The adverse effects of antiepileptic drugs can be divided into four categories

---

Adverse effects of all drugs, including antiepileptic drugs, can be divided – in an admittedly oversimplified way – into four fundamental groups. Each of these categories is relevant to the foregoing discussion (Principle 41) of single versus multiple drug therapy. In general, adverse effects are less likely with a single medication than with multiple drugs.

1. Dose-related adverse effects

A dose-related side effect occurs when the patient has received too much of the drug; it is, in effect, a mild overdose. Examples include double vision from carbamazepine, ataxia from phenytoin, sedation from phenobarbital, and tremor from valproate. The appropriate antidote is a lower dose. The single most important reason for maintaining patients on fewer medications is the difficulty of dealing with dose-related adverse effects. The patient is more likely, when on multiple medications, to have such effects for two reasons. First, the control of reasonable, nontoxic levels by the physician is clearly more difficult with multiple drugs than with a single medication; physicians vary in their ability to accomplish multi-drug regimens successfully. Secondly, some dose-related adverse effects are additive: ataxia may appear sooner with modest levels of carbamazepine combined with phenytoin than with either drug used singly at higher doses and levels.

2. Idiosyncratic adverse effects

Most idiosyncratic side effects occur within the first few months of therapy; some are severe and most require complete cessation of the medication. Examples include most skin rashes, bone marrow suppression, and hepatotoxicity. Because of greater patient exposure, the risk of such effects is clearly higher with multiple drugs than with single medications. However, little evidence exists for more than a simple additive effect; the idiosyncratic skin rash of phenobarbital, for example, is not more likely to occur in the presence of ethosuximide, which may also cause a rash. Unlike dose-related side effects (e.g., drowsiness or ataxia) in which the combination of drugs may cumulatively aggravate the toxicity, idiosyncratic reactions are usually related to a single medication.

Patients on multiple drugs who have an idiosyncratic reaction present the difficult problem of identifying which drug is the culprit. Because of the nature of idiosyncratic reactions, however, once a patient tolerates any drug for several months, the likelihood of an idiosyncratic reaction to that drug falls dramatically.

3. Drug interactions

The possibility of drug–drug interactions obviously increases with the number of medications. Furthermore, combinations of antiepileptic drugs may alter metabolism to produce changes in the levels of active and/or toxic metabolites; examples include the effect of phenytoin on carbamazepine and valproate on phenobarbital. Monotherapy with carbamazepine, for example, may yield well-tolerated plasma levels in the range of 14–16 μg/ml. When phenytoin is added in a multi-drug regimen, the maximal tolerated carbamazepine levels may be 8–10 μg/ml; although phenytoin increases carbamazepine metabolism, some carbamazepine dose reduction may be required. Likewise, phenytoin levels of 20–25 μg/ml or higher may be tolerated with monotherapy, but lower levels (and doses) are often necessary when phenytoin is combined with other drugs. Some of the newer antiepileptic drugs such as felbamate also interact with other drugs. Monotherapy eliminates these difficulties.

4. Teratogenicity

Little is known about the possible cumulative adverse effects of multiple drugs, either dose-related or idiosyncratic, on the developing fetus. For practical

PRINCIPLE 42

purposes, however, most agree that teratogenic effects are, at least in part, idiosyncratic effects and that epileptic women who are likely to become pregnant should take a minimum number of drugs. It has not been proven, however, that high doses of monotherapy are safer than moderate doses of multiple drugs. Is a high dose of phenytoin really safer for the fetus than moderate doses of phenytoin plus carbamazepine? Answers to such questions are not available from controlled studies or from inspection of available data.

---

43 The treatment of single seizures is controversial

A first seizure, particularly a generalized tonic–clonic seizure, can be a terrifying event. Most of the time no specific cause will be uncovered. Perhaps more unsettling, the neurologist will have to tell the patient that not only is there no explanation for the seizure, but it is very difficult to say whether there will be another.

Reported recurrence rates after single seizures vary from 30–70% over three years (Hauser *et al.*, 1982; Elwes *et al.*, 1985). The difference in the results of the studies may be due to inclusion of patients with different seizure types and etiologies, as well as patient sampling methods. Patients with an unambiguous etiology (other than an acute precipitant such as a transient metabolic dysfunction) are more likely to have recurrent seizures (Hauser *et al.*, 1982; Annegers *et al.*, 1985). Partial seizures are more likely to recur than generalized, children more likely than adults, and an abnormal EEG is probably an adverse prognostic factor (Hauser and Hesdorffer, 1990; Berg and Shinnar, 1991). Once two seizures have occurred, the probability of a third is very high (Hauser and Hesdorffer, 1990).

When a patient presents with a first generalized tonic–clonic seizure, several options have to be weighed. How bad will it be for the patient to have another seizure? Drug therapy can be expensive and associated with unpleasant side effects. Drugs reduce seizure frequency in patients with established seizure disorders, but can drugs prevent development of *epilepsy*?

Unfortunately there have been relatively few studies of the effect of drug therapy on recurrence after a single seizure. Camfield *et al.* (1989) reported that carbamazepine reduced recurrence after a nonfebrile partial or generalized tonic–clonic seizure in children, but that nearly one-third discontinued the drug due to side effects. A recent multi-center Italian study found that patients given phenytoin, phenobarbital, carbamazepine, or valproic acid after a first generalized tonic–clonic seizure were less likely in the following two years (18% *vs* 38%) to have a second (First Seizure Trial Group, 1993).

While single generalized tonic–clonic seizures are fairly common, isolated partial seizures are probably rare. Moreover the first event may not always be recognized, except in retrospect. It is hard to imagine that a single absence seizure would even be detected. Thus, it is reasonable to assume that a patient presenting with a 'first' partial or absence attack may already be suffering from recurrent spells.

44 Stopping antiepileptic drugs is a gamble

Patients who have become seizure-free often want to stop their AEDs. A number of prospective studies have been performed, and the chances of successful drug withdrawal can be estimated. Relapse rates in adults have been reported to range from 30–65% (Callaghan et al., 1988; Overweg et al., 1987). In a large multicenter randomized but unblinded study of patients who had been seizure-free for two years, 59% of those who stopped treatment, compared to 78% who did not, remained seizure-free for the subsequent two years (Medical Research Council Antiepileptic Drug Withdrawal Study Group, 1991).

Patients with more severe epilepsy – indicated by more frequent seizures or the need for multiple drugs before control – or with neurological deficits, or with a history of neurologic illness such as encephalitis, brain tumor, or metabolic disease, are less likely to remain seizure-free (Brorson and Wranne, 1987). Complex partial seizures may be an adverse risk factor, particularly if associated with secondary generalization (Callaghan et al., 1988). In adults, the EEG is a weak prognostic factor at best. The longer the seizure-free period before withdrawal, the greater the chance of success.

The prognosis for children appears to be better than for adults. Some studies suggest that as many as 75–90% will remain seizure free for several years after withdrawal (Emerson et al., 1981; Shinnar et al., 1985; Bouma et al., 1987; Arts et al., 1988; Matricardi et al., 1989). Shinnar et al. (1994) reported that seizures recurred in 36% during five years of follow-up; the children had been seizure-free for a mean of three years before drugs were stopped. In addition to the factors which predict recurrence in adults, an abnormal EEG (not necessarily showing epileptic discharges) before withdrawal is an adverse risk factor in most studies.

A meta-analysis of 25 studies suggested that risk of relapse at one year was 25% and at two years 29% (Berg and Shinnar, 1994). Patients with adolescent or adult-onset epilepsy had a higher chance of relapse. The prognosis for patients who remain seizure-free for two years is excellent, since most recurrences take place in that period (Thurston et al., 1982; Medical Research Council, 1991).

The patient most likely to stop drugs successfully has a normal neurologic exam, no history of CNS damage or disease, a normal EEG (if a child) and was easily controlled on a single drug after a few seizures. The risk of renewed seizures may vary from patient to patient, and is often thought to be lower in children. There is no evidence that children who relapse will be more difficult to control when drugs are restarted. Any child who has been seizure-free for two years and has no adverse risk factors should have a trial of drug withdrawal. Children with certain epileptic syndromes such as absence or juvenile myoclonic epilepsy, however, will often relapse when drugs are stopped.

For adults the choices are more nuanced, since the possibility of a seizure while driving or performing another skilled task has to be considered. Interestingly, in the Medical Research Council study, no overall group differences in psychosocial outcome could be detected between patients whose drugs were stopped and patients whose drugs were continued; the adverse effects of seizure recurrence apparently balanced the effect of continuing therapy (Jacoby *et al.*, 1992).

9 Therapy: Pharmacology and Pharmacokinetics

45	Give drugs after meals and at bedtime to maximize total daily intake without toxicity

From a pharmacokinetic point of view, the ideal way to give antiepileptic drugs is slow release into the bloodstream to achieve constant plasma (or brain) levels. Unfortunately, devices analogous to the insulin pump have not yet been developed for the treatment of seizures. In addition, many useful AEDs have no approved parenteral preparation or are poorly soluble in physiologic solutions.

Many AEDs have short half-lives, and multiple daily doses are necessary to ensure stable plasma levels. In addition, drugs with long half-lives, such as ethosuximide or the new AED felbamate, may cause gastrointestinal discomfort when the total daily dose is ingested at one time. For some drugs, there may be a limit to the rate of absorption, leading to reduced bioavailability for large doses. Thus the effect of even a long half-life drug may be enhanced, and toxicity reduced, by giving the drug in multiple doses.

Some studies have suggested that the absorption of amino-acid drugs like L-DOPA may be reduced when taken with a high-protein meal (Kurlan et al., 1988). Although this phenomenon has not yet been shown to affect AEDs, blood levels of the new drug gabapentin might conceivably be altered by this mechanism (Bialer, 1993).

Drug absorption may be highly variable, depending on the formulation (e.g., solution, coated tablet, or capsule), pH, and gastric emptying time, among other factors. Delayed gastric emptying, achlorhydria, or reduced small bowel surface area from previous surgery or from inflammatory bowel disease may reduce drug absorption (Welling, 1984). In the elderly, bowel motility and gastric emptying are reduced – while pH rises – potentially lowering drug absorption (Bender, 1968).

Differences in absorption have been suggested as a basis for case reports of neurologic toxicity or loss of seizure control due to substitution of generic for proprietary AEDs (Nuwer et al., 1990; Gilman et al., 1993). A double-blind trial showed therapeutic equivalence between Tegretol and one brand of generic carbamazepine (CBZ) (Oles et al., 1992). Several studies have suggested that overall steady-state phenytoin (PHT) levels do not change when patients are switched from Dilantin to generic PHT, but marked variability may exist among the generic drugs themselves (Petker and Morton, 1993; Soryal and Richens, 1992). Moreover, the bioavailability of Dilantin from the US appears to be significantly greater than the Dilantin from Taiwan (Tsai *et al.*, 1992). The problem of between-lot differences in bioavailability also may affect Tegretol as well as generic CBZ (Oles and Gal, 1993). Clinical problems, therefore, may be more likely to arise when a patient switches from one drug formulation to another rather than from branded to generic AEDs *per se.*

Patients who need maximal AED doses for seizure control will have better tolerability if a bedtime dose is included to make four daily doses. If the drug causes gastrointestinal (GI) distress, a bedtime snack may help. Hypnotic drugs like phenobarbital have traditionally been given at night. Although this may reduce the dose-related sedation, it may not change drug-related cognitive impairment.

Giving AEDs with meals may help to reduce GI distress as well as slow absorption and lead to smoother plasma levels. The total area under the plasma time-concentration curve is usually not changed, although peak levels may be lower (Theodore, 1990).

Unfortunately, AED compliance may be reduced by the need for the patient to remember to take the drugs several times a day. A number of methods can be used to help patients follow an AED regimen (Principle 50). Explaining to the patient that the drug being used has a short half-life and will work better when given more frequently is often helpful.

Some drugs have a long half-life. If the drug does not cause GI distress, some patients may do well on a once-a-day regimen. Others may find that taking the whole dose at once leads to undesirable neurologic side effects such as dizziness or diplopia. If a reliable formulation with 'smooth' release is not available, the drug is more likely to cause intermittent toxicity.

Another possible disadvantage of single daily dose regimens must be noted. Forgetting a single dose leads to the loss of an entire day's drug intake; a dangerous fall in blood levels may result.

46 The key to drug intake intervals is the drug's half-life

Drugs with a short half-life are cleared from the body faster than drugs with a long half-life and need to be given more frequently in order to maintain stable levels. After one half-life, only 50% of the administered drug remains in the body; after two, only 25%. Several antiepileptic drugs, such as valproic acid and carbamazepine, have half-lives of 12 hours or less in most clinical circumstances, and their levels may fluctuate dramatically during the day if given on a twice daily basis (Figure 46.1) (Rowan *et al.*, 1979). Excessive fluctuations in AED blood levels can have important therapeutic implications. Carbamazepine toxicity was significantly reduced when given four times a day when compared to twice daily dosing (Tomson, 1984). Clinical improvement has been reported when patients were switched from conventional to controlled release carbamazepine in a European trial (Bonneton *et al.*, 1993). An investigational slow-release valproic acid formulation has been reported to lead to decreased fluctuations in blood levels, reduced drug toxicity, and improved seizure control (Imaizumi *et al.*, 1992).

A number of factors which influence antiepileptic drug metabolism may need to be balanced by a change in dose or dosing interval. Most drugs are metabolized by the liver. Patients with hepatic disease, as well as the elderly, may have reduced metabolism and be more susceptible to antiepileptic drug toxicity (Cloyd, 1991). The elimination of antiepileptic drugs can be affected by pharmacologic interactions as well as physiologic alterations. Hepatic enzyme inducers such as phenobarbital, phenytoin, or carbamazepine, usually reduce the levels of co-administered drugs. However, interactions may be complex. Phenobarbital, for example, may occasionally raise phenytoin levels rather than lower them because it competes for its metabolism with the same enzyme systems. Phenytoin

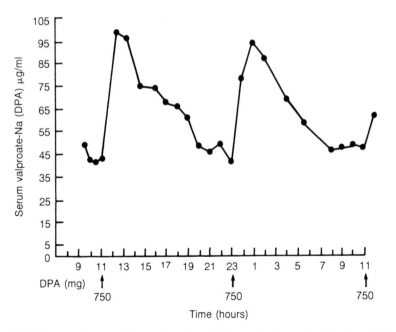

Figure 46.1 Serum valproate fluctuations in a 12-hour dosing schedule (modified from Rowan *et al.*, 1979), with permission.

PRINCIPLE 46

induces conversion of primidone to phenobarbital and phenylethylmalonamide, but blocks metabolism of phenobarbital, leading to a marked rise in phenobarbital levels (Porro et al., 1982). The expected plasma half-lives and time to steady state for the classical antiepileptic drugs are listed in Table 46.1.

Drug 'interactions' may even occur when only one antiepileptic drug is being given. Carbamazepine (CBZ), for example, induces its own metabolism – a process which may take 3–4 weeks after the drug is started (Bertilsson et al., 1980). Carbamazepine levels may fall, and seizures continue even though the patient is taking a steady dose which originally produced a therapeutic level.

Antiepileptic drugs can interact with other drugs, such as oral contraceptives or anticoagulants. Increased oral contraceptive metabolism has led to unexpected pregnancy (Kutt, 1989). Table 46.2 shows the major clinically significant drug interactions. There may be considerable interindividual variability in the extent of interactions, just as in drug absorption, protein binding, and metabolism. Additional factors complicate the prediction of clinical effects. Increased metabolism of parent drugs may produce new metabolites which themselves may be active. Drug interactions can change binding to plasma proteins, leading to altered clearance.

Some of the newer antiepileptic drugs are excreted unchanged by the kidney. Although not affected by hepatic enzyme induction, their levels may be affected – and doses need to be reduced – in patients with renal disease or in the elderly; the latter have reduced renal plasma flow and creatinine clearance.

Table 46.1 Plasma half-life of six antiepileptic drugs

Drug	Half-life*	Time to reach steady state
Carbamazepine	12 hours	3 days
Valproate	12 hours	3 days
Primidone**	12 hours	3 days
Phenytoin	1 day	5 days***
Ethosuximide	2 days	10 days
Phenobarbital	4 days	3 weeks

*Half-life is usually shorter when the drug is coadministered with enzyme-inducing drugs (including some other antiepileptic drugs). Half-life may be longer at onset of administration (especially with carbamazepine).
**Primidone is converted rapidly to phenobarbital (Principle 84).
***Phenytoin obeys saturation kinetics (Principle 58).
Modified from Penry and Newmark (1979), with permission.

Table 46.2 Clinically significant antiepileptic drug interactions

Drug	Levels increased by	Levels decreased by	Increases levels	Decreases levels
PHT	PB, FBM, isoniazid, rifampin, sulfa drugs cimetidine	PB, VPA, CBZ	PB	narcotics steroids theophylline dicumarol, CBZ, VPA
CBZ	PHT, erythromycin cimetidine, verapamil	VPA, PHT, PB	PHT	VPA, ETHO, PHT, haldol
CBZ-E	VPA, PHT, PB			
PB	PHT, VPA	phenothiazine		narcotics steroids dicumarol, theophylline VPA, PHT, CBZ, cimetidine
VPA		PB, PHT, CBZ	PB, PHT, ETHO, CBZ-E	
ETHO	VPA	CBZ		

PB = phenobarbital; PHT = phenytoin; ETHO = ethosuximide CBZ = carbamazepine; CBZ-E = carbamazepine epoxide; VPA = valproic acid; FBM = felbamate.

---

47 The time needed to reach a new steady-state plasma drug level is not determined by the amount of the dose change

Short half-life drugs have the advantage that their levels can be adjusted more quickly. After a change in dose, it takes about five half-lives for a new steady-state level to be reached. Only 2 to 3 days are needed to evaluate the effect of a carbamazepine dose change, compared to 5 to 7 days for phenytoin (Figure 47.1). Waiting for the new steady state to assess seizure control is more important than waiting for toxicity, since side effects are not likely to go away while blood levels continue to rise, but the full effect of a dose increase on seizure frequency may be delayed. Dose-related drug toxicity can be minimized by making small increments in dose, particularly when patients are already taking

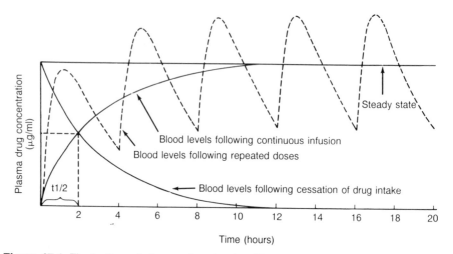

Figure 47.1 Fluctuation of plasma drug levels with repeated drug administration (dotted lines). The steady-state level after 5–7 half-lives approaches that achieved by continuous infusion. In this case, the half-life of the drug is only 2 hours (from Porter, 1981).

high AED doses. It can take a long time to evaluate fully the effect of even small changes in drug doses.

Several computer algorithms have been developed, particularly for phenytoin dosing in healthy outpatients (Privitera, 1993). The steady-state level is a function of the dose, fraction absorbed, dosing interval, and clearance (Theodore, 1990). Only two of these parameters (dose and dosing interval) can be controlled by the physician. Clearance, for example, is the total rate of drug removal from the body – by hepatic, renal, or other routes – and can be affected by pathological and physiological alterations. Because these variables are difficult to quantify, steady-state levels are difficult to predict. Obtaining frequent reports of seizure occurence and toxicity, as well as blood levels, may be necessary as a substitute.

Patients can be given a loading dose in order to hasten the full therapeutic effect of a long-half-life drug, e.g., the administration of intravenous phenytoin for status epilepticus. Since phenytoin has good GI absorption, patients who are not in status can be given an oral loading dose if rapid achievement of a therapeutic level is desirable. Giving 300–400 mg every 4 hours is often better tolerated than giving the whole dose at once.

48 Plasma drug levels are only a guide

The central role of antiepileptic drug level measurement in clinical management is dictated by the peculiarly intermittent nature of seizures. Patients may go for weeks or months without any clinical signs or symptoms against which drug effects can be judged. Physicians rarely see seizures occur, the neurological examination is usually normal, and clinical signs – such as nystagmus – are not only inconsistently related but are unreliable guides to the desired or undesirable drug effects.

The primary use of AED levels is to determine whether the patient is protected from seizures during the time when attacks are not occurring. Since the 1960s, a large number of clinical studies have been performed in an attempt to relate AED levels to seizure control and drug toxicity (Theodore, 1992), and broad general guidelines have been established (Table 48.1). Unfortunately, many studies of AED therapeutic ranges have suffered from design flaws which complicate their interpretation. (It is particularly difficult to evaluate the relation of drug levels to clinical effect when patients are taking more than one drug.) Blood levels are based on population data, and do not always apply to individual patients, who may tolerate AED levels, particularly PHT and CBZ, considerably beyond the 'therapeutic range'. One should not hesitate to use doses which produce such levels, particularly with monotherapy, if clinically indicated (Lesser *et al.*, 1984; Schmidt, 1983).

Although AED levels are frequently measured, it is uncertain how much effect such results have on clinical seizure management. Neurologists themselves disagree on the limits for the therapeutic ranges, not to mention what to do with the results (Dooley *et al.*, 1993). In an outpatient clinic setting, only 29% of the levels above the therapeutic range were followed by a change in regimen; in 20% of these cases, the dose was raised (Larkin *et al.*, 1991).

Table 48.1 Therapeutic levels (mg/l) of standard antiepileptic drugs

Drug	Effective level	High effective level*	Toxic level
Carbamazepine	6–15	12	>8
Phenytoin	10–20	18	>15
Phenobarbital	10–30	25	>20
Primidone	5–15	12	>10
Valproic acid	50–100	80	>100
Ethosuximide	50–100	80	>100

*Minimum levels that should be reached (particularly during monotherapy) in patients with refractory seizures before deciding the drug has failed to help. Higher levels are often possible with monotherapy. Levels are trough levels drawn before the morning medication.

Standardizing the time of day at which AED levels are drawn is most important, and the most consistent and useful data are obtained from trough morning samples. If possible, epilepsy clinics should be held in the morning so patients can come in for trough levels without an extra trip. Levels obtained at a fixed post-dose interval later in the day may be affected by diurnal variation in absorption and metabolism, as well by as the effects of food.

Levels drawn at different times can be used for different therapeutic judgements, particularly when short half-life drugs such as CBZ and VPA are being used. Trough levels assess the 'safety net' for seizure protection; peak measurements – or even better, measurements at the time the patient is having symptoms – best evaluate drug toxicity. Ideally, several levels should be obtained throughout the course of the day. Confusion of antiepileptic drug toxicity with other signs and symptoms must be avoided. Simple partial seizures, for example, may cause symptoms such as dizziness – which could also be due to drug toxicity. If AED levels are low, toxicity is less likely.

Clinical drug toxicity usually can be detected by the examining physician; in the pre-AED plasma level era, Yahr *et al.* (1952) suggested that AED therapy should be 'pushed' to toxicity before a drug is 'given up'. However, AED levels can help assess risk for toxicity, especially more subtle – particularly neuropsychological – toxicity, which all antiepileptic drugs may produce at high levels (Dodrill and Troupin, 1991) (Principle 98).

If a patient is seizure-free on an AED dose which does not produce any side effects, why should levels be measured? Usually, it is not helpful to raise the dose of seizure-free patients with 'subtherapeutic' levels (Woo *et al.*, 1988). Compliance, however, can decrease over time; perhaps the patient has really been seizure-free – and no drug is needed.

---

49 **A reliable clinical laboratory is critical for accurate monitoring of plasma drug levels, particularly of unbound drug levels and metabolites**

Any laboratory which measures antiepileptic drugs should take part in one of the proficiency testing programs run by the American Association for Clinical Chemistry, Washington, DC, or the American College of Pathologists, Skokie, Illinois. Participation in such a program improves the accuracy of laboratory performance dramatically (Pippenger *et al.*, 1977).

Methods for antiepileptic drug measurement include gas and high pressure liquid chromatography, enzyme multiplied immunochemical assay (EMIT), fluorescence polarization immunoassay, noninstrumented enzyme immunoassay, and other techniques (Kupferberg, 1978; Jolley et al., 1981; Schottelius, 1978; Zuk et al., 1985). Chromatographic methods allow simultaneous determination of multiple drug levels, and may be somewhat more accurate for research purposes, but the immunoassays are convenient, cheaper, and more widely used clinically. For practical purposes, there is excellent correlation among the various methods (Cochran et al., 1990; Thomas et al., 1991).

Free drug levels can be measured after using ultrafiltration or equilibrium dialysis to separate the drug from plasma protein. The temperature at which the procedure is performed can affect the results, since binding is greater at room temperature (25°C) than body temperature.

Theoretically, only unbound drug reaches sites of physiologic action. Protein binding can be decreased by reduction in serum albumin (the major plasma binding protein), pregnancy, hepatic or renal disease, or competition for binding sites by substances such as fatty acids or other drugs (Theodore, 1987). Alpha$_1$-acid glycoprotein and lipoproteins, which are elevated in acute illness, can transiently increase the binding of basic drugs such as carbamazepine (Piafsky, 1980). Decreased binding increases drug clearance: total drug level is decreased, free fraction increases, but free level should remain stable. The more tightly bound a drug, the greater effect a small alteration in binding will have on its free fraction (Table 49.1).

Usually, there is an excellent correlation between free and total AED levels, and no clinical advantage in measuring the former (Theodore, 1987). It may be valuable to measure free phenytoin levels or valproic acid levels when altered binding is likely (Booker and Darcy, 1973; Theodore et al., 1985a; Peterson et al., 1991; Lenn and Robertson, 1992). Because the normal free fraction is greater for carbamazepine and phenobarbital, free levels are less likely to be significantly affected by changes in binding.

Unbound antiepileptic drug levels can also be measured in saliva; venipuncture is thereby avoided. Although the method has many technical pitfalls, it may be particularly useful for children (Schramm et al., 1991).

In some clinical situations, measurement of carbamazepine-10,11-epoxide (the active metabolite of carbamazepine), which has anticonvulsant activity and side effects similar to carbamazepine itself, may be helpful (Eadie, 1991). Epoxide

Table 49.1 Antiepileptic drug protein binding

Drug	Free fraction	Interactions
Phenytoin	10–15%	VPA increases
Phenobarbital	50%	
Valproic acid	5–15%	PHT increases
Carbamazepine	25–40%	
CBZ-10, 11-epoxide	50%	

levels, usually 20–25% of parent drug, are increased by high carbamazepine levels, or by other antiepileptic drugs such as phenytoin or valproic acid (Theodore *et al.*, 1989a). Phenobarbital increases both carbamazepine-epoxide clearance and conversion of parent drug to metabolite (Spina *et al.*, 1991). Since the carbamazepine-epoxide free fraction is greater than carbamazepine itself, the relative effect of increased epoxide levels may be enhanced. This phenomenon can explain the unusual but paradoxical observation of increased carbamazepine toxicity when the parent drug levels are falling.

---

50 Noncompliance is a common cause of uncontrolled seizures

Poor compliance with antiepileptic drugs may occur in 30–50% of patients at some time (Leppik, 1988). The problem may range from occasional confusion or omission of doses in a complex regimen to sudden cessation of all drug intake. Noncompliance may be intermittent or episodic and may be related to significant external life events or stresses. Patients may comply with some aspects of treatment; they may, for example, take all their drugs but never appear for appointments or blood levels – and then call to have a prescription refilled by phone. Others may continuously adjust their own doses (perhaps as well or better than their neurologist!), indulge in behaviors thought inimical to good seizure control such as imbibing alcoholic beverages all night, or even deliberately be noncompliant (Figure 50.1).

Since noncompliance with drug doses usually is intermittent, it is likely to be reflected by fluctuating levels on a stable regimen, whereas consistently low levels are usually caused by poor absorption, reduced protein binding, rapid metabolism, or other pharmacologic variables. Increasing drug doses in the face of noncompliance can lead to the rapid onset of toxicity when the patient suddenly decides to start taking drugs as directed. In well-monitored patients, the coefficient of variation (standard deviation of the plasma concentration divided by the mean) should be less than 20% (Leppik, 1988).

Noncompliance may be voluntary or involuntary. Patients may be unable to understand their drug regimen because of neuropsychological impairment, or they may be unable to afford their drugs or the cost of appointments. In patients taking phenytoin or theophylline, the most common cause of noncompliance, irrespective of education, was failure to understand the need to take medication regularly (Dowse and Futter, 1991). In some cases, the fear of changes in regimen or of new drugs may influence compliance. Assertion of autonomy and independence, particularly for young adults (Figure 50.2), may be a significant factor in

FEMALE 26 YEARS

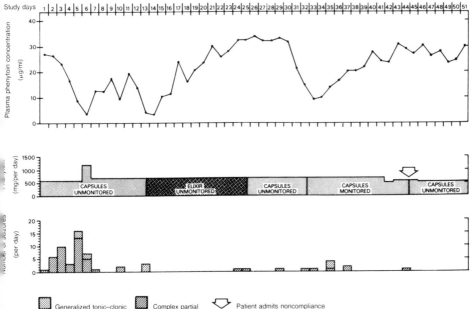

Figure 50.1 Graphic representation of plasma phenytoin concentration and phenytoin dosage in relation to number of seizures in a hospitalized 26-year-old woman with deliberate noncompliance. During days 1–13, she had many seizures and erratic levels; capsules were unmonitored. During days 14–25, she was given phenytoin elixir; plasma drug levels rose and seizure control improved dramatically. On day 26 she was again started on phenytoin capsules unmonitored; the levels fell and seizures recurred. On day 33, the patient's mouth was inspected with each (daily) phenytoin dose. The levels again rose and seizures abated. On day 45, she admitted throwing the medicine into the commode. She was discharged with excellent seizure control, but one year later we received a long-distance phone call from a physician with a fascinating patient (the same) who could not absorb phenytoin! (from Desai *et al.*, 1978, with permission).

refusal to follow a physician's instructions (Taylor, 1993). Occasional patients may derive 'secondary gain' – such as disability payments or a caregiver's continuous attention – from persistent seizures.

A number of approaches may improve compliance. Increasing the frequency of clinic visits, whether the patient sees a physician or nonphysician, may be effective (Wannamaker *et al.*, 1980). Simplification of dosing regimens is desirable, but the effect of missing an entire day's drug in a once daily regimen may outweigh the hoped-for increase in compliance. A long drug half-life mitigates the effect of a missed dose, so long as the drug does not have a steep concentration-effect curve – in which case a small fall in blood level will lead to a marked drop in antiepileptic potency (Levy, 1993).

Education about the need to take drugs regularly should include family

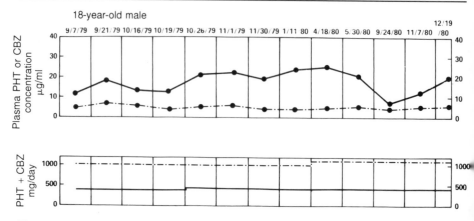

Figure 50.2 The 18-year-old son of a prominent scientist had gradually increasing doses and plasma levels of phenytoin (solid line) and carbamazepine (dotted line), which correlated with improved control of his complex partial seizures until he left home for college in September 1980. On September 19 and 20, he had several secondarily generalized tonic–clonic seizures in the college dormitory. He was taken home on September 21, and blood drug levels were determined 3 days later on September 24. The phenytoin (PHT) level had fallen dramatically from the level in May 1980, but the carbamazepine (CBZ) was apparently unchanged. This puzzling observation was explained by the parents' careful monitoring of drug intake during the patient's 3 days at home. Carbamazepine, with a short half-life, returned quickly to a steady state, and by September 24, the level was again therapeutic. Phenytoin, however, with a relatively long half-life, took much longer to return to steady state, and the September 24 level was therefore low. Seizure control returned after drug intake was resumed.

members or other caregivers. Patients can be asked to recite their drug schedule at each visit, reinforcing the need for consistency. Patients can be encouraged to count out each day's dose in the morning, placing the pills in a divided container. Pill-containers with built-in alarms are now becoming available, at least for clinical trials (Cramer and Russell, 1988). Most important is to try to understand each patient's reason for noncompliance and to approach the problem on an individual basis.

10 Therapy: Partial Seizures

---

51 Use carbamazepine or phenytoin for partial seizures

Among the drugs, both old and new, which have been shown to be effective for complex partial seizures, carbamazepine and phenytoin still offer the best combination of efficacy and low toxicity. In a randomized prospective trial of 622 patients, the Veterans' Administration Cooperative Study compared carbamazepine, phenytoin, primidone and phenobarbital (Mattson et al., 1985). Over three years, treatment with carbamazepine or phenytoin was significantly more likely to be successful than phenobarbital or primidone. Most treatment failures were caused by a combination of toxicity and poor seizure control; more patients failed due to the former alone than the latter alone. Comparing seizure control alone, the four drugs were equivalent for generalized tonic–clonic seizures, but carbamazepine was superior to phenobarbital or primidone for complex partial seizures; phenytoin was intermediate. Some 65% of patients had complete control of partial seizures on carbamazepine at 12 months.

In a subsequent study of 480 patients, the same group of investigators compared carbamazepine with valproic acid (Mattson et al., 1992). Valproic acid was as effective for generalized tonic–clonic seizure control, but carbamazepine led to fewer complex partial seizures (0.9 vs 2.2 per month) and was associated with less toxicity. Other investigators had reported no differences among phenytoin, carbamazepine, and valproic acid for complex partial seizures, perhaps because their patient populations were too small to detect the small differences between drugs in efficacy and toxicity (Turnbull et al., 1982; Callaghan et al., 1985). Bruni and Albright (1983) reported that the response of patients with partial seizures to valproic acid tended to diminish over time.

The choice between carbamazepine and phenytoin can be based on patient preference, which will usually depend on the difference in side effects. Since phenytoin causes hirsutism, carbamazepine is probably a better choice for women. The two drugs have comparable neuropsychological toxicity (Meador et al., 1990; Dodrill and Troupin, 1991). Phenytoin is cheaper, and has a longer half-life.

About 40% of patients who do not have acceptable seizure control on one drug will have significant improvement – and 10% become seizure-free – on a combination of carbamazepine and phenytoin or other appropriate combinations (Schmidt, 1982; Callaghan *et al.*, 1985; Mattson *et al.*, 1985). The increased seizure control is not without price, as adverse drug effects are increased with drug combinations. Three-drug combinations rarely confer sufficient benefit to justify the increased toxicity.

Valproic acid or one of the newer antiepileptic drugs (see Chapter 11) should be tried if patients do not respond to, or cannot tolerate, carbamazepine and phenytoin. Although barbiturates may be equally effective for seizure control, their neuropsychological toxicity limits their utility unless other approaches are contraindicated.

Several older antiepileptic drugs have been tried for complex partial seizures, but the recent introduction of so many new alternatives will make their use very rare. Methsuximide is a relative of the antiabsence drug ethosuximide, but has greater toxicity. It blocks the metabolism of phenytoin and phenobarbital, which could have accounted for part of the therapeutic effect in some trials (Wilder and Buchanan, 1981; Browne *et al.*, 1983). Mephenytoin is metabolized to the sedative drug nirvanol (Theodore *et al.*, 1984b). Although mephenytoin does not cause hirsutism or gingival hyperplasia, it shares phenytoin's neurologic side effects of nystagmus, diplopia and ataxia (Troupin *et al.*, 1976). More important, nirvanol is associated with a high incidence of blood dyscrasias. Phenacemide, another phenytoin analogue, is associated with a high incidence of toxicity and is almost never used.

---

52 A 1000 mg daily dose of carbamazepine is often not enough for an adult

---

The therapeutic range often given for carbamazepine, 4–12 mg/l, is often too low. Many patients tolerate much higher levels without toxicity (Kutt *et al.*, 1975; Monaco *et al.*, 1976; Simonsen *et al.*, 1976; Troupin *et al.*, 1977). Many patients on doses of 800–1000 mg/day will have a trough morning level of only 4–5 mg/l, which is probably not enough to provide adequate protection against complex partial seizures. To achieve therapeutic blood levels, many patients take 1400–1600 mg/day; some may need doses as high as 2000 mg/day.

Carbamazepine should be started at a relatively low dose, 300–400 mg/day, to reduce initial gastrointestinal and CNS adverse effects. Increases of 200 mg/week should be well-tolerated. However, autoinduction of metabolism will occur over the first 3–4 weeks of therapy, and drug levels will fall. A gradual increase in the dose usually is necessary. The optimal dose for each patient will take 1–2 months to establish. It is important not to be discouraged by early side effects and to warn patients that a period of dose adjustment will be necessary.

The shorter half-life of carbamazepine – compared to PB and PHT – means that greater fluctuations will occur throughout the day. The relation between these fluctuations and drug toxicity is uncertain, but they can be reduced by giving the drug in three or four doses (Tomson, 1984; Reinvang et al., 1991). Although a controlled release form of carbamazepine is undergoing tests in Europe, it may not offer significant advantages in terms of reducing toxicity (Aldenkamp et al., 1987; Bonneton et al., 1993).

CBZ has an active metabolite, carbamazepine 10,11-epoxide (CBZ-E), which may contribute to the therapeutic effect of the drug (Eichelbaum et al., 1976). CBZ metabolism is usually increased by coadministration of other AEDs, during which the CBZ-E/CBZ ratio increases (Brodie et al., 1983; Theodore et al., 1989a). Measurement of CBZ-E, however, has not been shown to be clinically useful (Theodore et al., 1989a). CBZ binds to plasma proteins less than does PHT and is less likely to have relevant free level effects (Theodore, 1987). No convincing relation between CBZ free levels and toxicity or seizure control has been demonstrated (Lesser et al., 1984).

---

53   **Increase the carbamazepine dose in 100 mg increments after a 1200 mg daily dose has been achieved**

When patients are near the upper limit of their own 'therapeutic range', small increases in carbamazepine levels may lead to marked increases in toxicity and doses should be increased by only 100 mg/day. Some brands of carbamazepine are scored 200 mg tablets and can be broken in half; alternatively, the 100 mg chewable form can be used.

Dose adjustments should also be made *less frequently* at the upper dose ranges – perhaps every 1–2 weeks. More care may be needed when patients are taking carbamazepine with other drugs.

When patients report adverse drug effects, the physician should find out exactly when they occur and how long they last. Often, rearrangement of doses can eliminate them without lowering total drug intake and endangering seizure control.

Alterations in drug metabolism during childhood are related to maturational processes, and cannot be predicted from weight gain alone (Albani et al., 1992). The greatest fall in the carbamazepine plasma level/dose ratio occurs from age 9–12, and monitoring should be more careful during this period.

In the elderly, slow and careful adjustments of carbamazepine dose are particularly important. Although some studies suggest that elderly patients may metabolize carbamazepine more rapidly – and need higher doses for therapeutic blood levels – these patients tend to be more sensitive to AED side effects (Leppik, 1992). Loss of balance can lead to falls with serious consequences such as hip fracture. Even relatively mild hyponatremia may cause confusion in the elderly.

---

54 Diplopia is the most common dose-related side effect of high plasma carbamazepine levels

---

As many as 50% of patients will report some adverse drug effect during their treatment with carbamazepine, but only 5% will need to stop the drug for this reason (Pellock, 1987; Gram and Jensen, 1989). Moreover, side effects are more frequent when patients are taking other drugs in addition to carbamazepine (Hoeppener et al., 1980; Pellock, 1987). Ataxia tends to occur at higher blood levels than diplopia; patients may have mild abnormalities of tandem gait without awareness of any gait problems. Drowsiness is most common on initiation of therapy and is nearly always transient; headache may also occur. Patients may complain of nonspecific blurred vision which, unlike true diplopia, does not go away when one eye is covered. (True monocular diplopia occurs in the context of eye disease, or occipitoparietal dysfunction.) Gastrointestinal disturbances are reported by only 5–10% of patients.

Hyponatremia, which is usually asymptomatic, can occur in up to one-third of patients; it is more common in the elderly and is observed especially at high doses (Gram and Jensen, 1989). Decreased serum sodium may, at least theoretically, increase seizures or contribute to side effects such as dizziness, drowsiness, or headache. Although hyponatremia usually responds to fluid restriction, this may not be practical on a chronic basis and the carbamazepine dose may have to be reduced.

Since carbamazepine has a relatively short half-life, dose related side effects are often transient – lasting 30 minutes to 2 hours – and are related to the time of drug ingestion. Rearranging doses, and particularly giving smaller, more frequent doses, may reduce toxicity by maintaining more constant plasma levels. If a patient has toxicity while taking more than one drug, the blood levels should be obtained at the time the symptoms occur in order to identify the offending drug – which may not be the drug most recently started or increased. Carbamazepine epoxide levels may also be obtained, but their clinical interpretation is uncertain (Theodore et al., 1989a). Although complaints of side effects are rare at blood levels below 8 mg/l, many patients can tolerate much higher levels, particularly when taking carbamazepine alone (Hoeppener *et al.*, 1980).

Occasional patients, especially those with significant neurologic disease – and with cognitive and motor impairment in addition to their seizures – develop choreoathetosis or dystonia on high carbamazepine doses. Rarely, acute psychoses have been precipitated. Exacerbation of atonic seizures has been reported, particularly in children with static encephalopathy and slow-spike wave on EEG (Pellock, 1987). This observation, however, has not been tested in a controlled study.

---

55 The most important idiosyncratic side effect of carbamazepine is hematologic

---

Bone marrow depression caused by carbamazepine therapy is rare, estimated to occur in 0.5 cases per 100,000 treatment years (Hart and Easton, 1982). Aplastic anemia may be slightly more common than agranulocytosis. Unfortunately, when these complications occur, they are fatal in 30–50% of patients (Gram and Jensen, 1989). Although many of the first cases occurred in older patients who had taken the drug for trigeminal neuralgia, the small total number of cases reported makes it difficult to conclude that the elderly are truly more sensitive.

Transient, or persistent but nonprogressive, leukopenia occurs in up to 10% of patients (Hart and Easton, 1982). Patients with white counts below 3000/ml^3 can remain on carbamazepine as long as they need the drug for seizure control. Reducing the dose may help, but counts can fluctuate up and down while carbamazepine intake is unchanged. It may be more important to follow the absolute neutrophil count; infection is more likely when counts fall below 1000 (1×10^9/l), and particularly below 500 (Bagby, 1988).

The evidence does not support obtaining blood counts more frequently in patients taking carbamazepine than other antiepileptic drugs. For convenience, patients on chronic therapy can have a complete blood count (CBC) whenever their antiepileptic drug levels are measured.

Like all other drugs, carbamazepine is associated with occasional elevation of liver function tests (Pellock, 1987). Some enzyme assays, particularly the gamma-glutamyl transpeptidase, merely reflect induction of hepatic activity, and have little clinical significance. Liver function tests should be elevated to at least twice normal before a dose reduction is considered. Carbamazepine-induced hepatitis can occur in the context of a generalized hypersensitivity reaction, accompanied by fever, rash, and granulomata seen on liver biopsy (Levy *et al.*, 1981).

Carbamazepine-induced rashes, reported in 3–16% of patients exposed, are usually mild, but it is prudent to stop the drug and try something else; 5–10% of patients with rashes have more severe involvement such as exfoliative dermatitis (Pellock 1987; Pelekanos et al., 1991). Unfortunately, patients who react to one drug are more likely to react to another, particularly if the two drugs are structurally similar. In a patient has had a rash on carbamazepine, one of the new drugs may be tried (see Chapter 11). Some patients who had an allergic reaction to carbamazepine have been able to tolerate oxcarbazepine.

Antiepileptic drugs, particularly phenytoin, phenobarbital, and carbamazepine, can interfere with thyroid function by displacing T4 from plasma protein binding sites, as well as increasing both conversion to T3 and the clearance of the unbound hormone (Liewendahl et al., 1978; Isojarvi et al., 1992). Most of the time a new steady-state is established, patients are clinically euthyroid, and the thyroid stimulating hormone (TSH) is normal. If hypothyroidism is suspected, a thyrotropin releasing factor (TRF) stimulation test can be performed to check for heightened pituitary responsiveness. Other potential endocrine effects of carbamazepine include reduction in free testosterone levels, which may be related to sexual dysfunction; occasional patients do, in fact, report impotence (Dana-Haeri et al., 1982). Carbamazepine seems to interfere less than phenytoin or phenobarbital with vitamin D and calcium metabolism (Gram and Jensen, 1989).

Increases in total and high density lipoprotein (HDL) cholesterol in patients taking carbamazepine have been reported (Isojarvi et al., 1993). Transient increases are also observed in low density lipoprotein (LDL) cholesterol and triglycerides; the clinical significance of these increases is unknown.

Carbamazepine, like its relatives, the tricyclic antidepressants, can cause bradycardia (Gram and Jensen, 1989). The elderly may be more sensitive to this side effect; Stokes–Adams attacks have been reported.

Since its introduction, carbamazepine has proved to be one of the safest and best tolerated of the antiepileptic drugs.

---

56 A 300 mg daily dose of phenytoin is often not enough for an adult

Phenytoin comes in 100 mg capsules; most patients can tolerate three pills per day very well, but many eventually become toxic on four. Unfortunately, the smaller dose is not enough to reliably provide therapeutic serum levels. Buchthal and Svensmark (1959–1960), in a landmark investigation, studied the relation of serum PHT levels to clinical effect. The lowest level at which they thought efficacy occurred was 10 mg/l, but seizure control was more likely with levels above 15 mg/l, and some of their patients tolerated levels as high as 50 mg/l (Buchthal and Svensmark, 1959–1960). In ambulatory patients with generalized tonic–clonic seizures, greater improvement was found when PHT levels were in the 15–20 mg/l than in the 10–15 mg/l range (Buchthal et al., 1960).

The 'therapeutic blood level' for phenytoin depends on both seizure type and severity of the epileptic syndrome. Schmidt et al. (1986) found that patients with persistent seizures referred to an epilepsy clinic who had GTCS alone were well-controlled at a mean PHT level of 14 mg/l, while those who had complex partial seizures (CPS) needed a mean of 23 mg/l. On the other hand, adults with newly diagnosed epilepsy needed a blood level of only 6.8 ± 2.7 mg/l for seizure control. In interpreting the efficacy of the phenytoin levels in this study however, it is important to remember that many of the patients had had only a single seizure; less than half of these patients would be expected to have a second attack in the two year period, even without treatment (Principle 43). Interestingly, their dose was 4.9 ± 1.7 mg/kg; some patients needed more than 400 mg/day even to maintain plasma levels near 10 mg/l.

Because phenytoin has a long half-life, an oral loading dose should be used if it is necessary to obtain therapeutic levels rapidly without intravenous administration (discussed in Principle 83). Usually, patients will tolerate 15–20 mg/kg given over several hours (Wilder et al., 1973).

---

57 Phenytoin doses should be increased in small increments

Increases in phenytoin dose from, for example, 300 to 400 mg per day, can lead eventually to much larger changes in drug levels than occurred after an increase of 200 to 300 mg/day (Principle 58). The delayed appearance of drug toxicity after a dose change can be confusing and frustrating. Luckily, phenytoin is available in smaller dosage forms which can be used for more accurate titration.

In addition to the 100 mg capsule, phenytoin comes in a 30 mg capsule, and a 50 mg chewable tablet, which has a different formulation. The capsules contain the sodium salt of phenytoin (often called 'diphenylhydantoin sodium' in older literature). The chewable tablet phenytoin formulation is the free acid. It contains 8% more phenytoin per mg, so the 50 mg tablet is equivalent to 54 mg of the capsules. Small differences in the rate of absorption between the formulations are not clinically significant as both are nearly completely bioavailable.

Since most patients need a daily dose of about 5 mg/kg to obtain therapeutic phenytoin blood levels, a substantial number of patients need a dose between 300 and 400 mg. Either the chewable tablets or the 30 mg capsules can be used, but the latter do not have to be broken in half to obtain the smaller increments.

58 Watch for saturation kinetics with phenytoin

Phenytoin is almost completely metabolized before renal excretion. The most important step (responsible for 70–90% of phenytoin metabolites) in the pathway, hydroxylation to 5-(4-hydoxyphenyl)-5-phenylhydantoin, is catalyzed by arene oxidase, a saturable enzyme. Its activity can also be blocked by carbamazepine (Browne *et al.*, 1988). In addition, a small number of patients inherit a tendency to metabolize phenytoin more slowly than normal and may become toxic on low doses (Glazko *et al.*, 1982).

The Michaelis–Menton equation (Albert Michaelis was a famous German chemist who came to the United States in 1926; Maud Menton, the first woman medical student at the University of Toronto, eventually became Professor of Pathology at the University of Pittsburgh) describes the rate of an enzyme-catalyzed chemical reaction (Gjedde, 1989). V*max* is the maximum velocity, and K*m* the substrate (or drug) concentration when velocity is half of the maximum rate. Steady state concentration, Css, is equal to $RKm/(Vmax - R)$, where R is the dosing rate. Phenytoin is the only antiepileptic drug affected by saturation of metabolism, since it has therapeutic plasma levels higher than its K*m* (mean 6.2 mg/l), and a dosing rate greater than 10% of V*max* (Browne and Chang Sun, 1989).

When metabolism is at or near saturation, small changes in dose (either up or down) may lead to very large changes in level (Figure 58.1). Moreover, the effect of the change on toxicity and seizure control may not be immediately apparent, as up to a month may be required – punctuated by false plateaus – for a new steady-state to be established (Theodore *et al.*, 1984a). Dose increases need to be small and should be separated by enough time to fully observe the impact of the increase; indeed, phenytoin levels may increase for a very long time after an increase in dose.

Marked interindividual variability in K*m* and V*max* makes difficult the prediction of when metabolism will begin to be saturated in a particular patient. Some patients need 500 mg/day; others cannot tolerate more than 150. Based on computer simulations and Bayesian forecasting, Privitera (1993) suggested increasing the dose by 50 mg/day if the plasma concentration is below 12 mg/l, and by 30 mg/day if the concentration is higher. Following these rules, the plasma phenytoin level was always maintained below 25 mg/l. However, patients vary in their sensitivity, and clinical signs and plasma levels should be monitored closely. Phenytoin V*max* is higher in children than adults, accounting for its shorter half-life and the need for proportionately higher doses to achieve therapeutic levels (Eadie *et al.*, 1976).

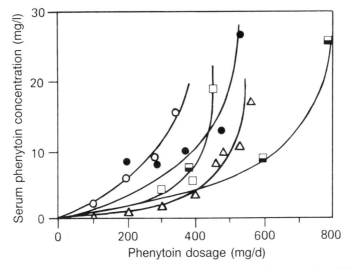

Figure 58.1 Nonlinear effect of phenytoin dose on plasma phenytoin level. Five patients received increasing oral doses of phenytoin, and the steady-state level was measured at each dose. As expected from saturation kinetics, the curves are not linear: as the dose increases, the plasma phenytoin levels rise at an even more rapid rate. The patients showed marked variation in the plasma phenytoin levels achieved at the various doses (from Porter and Pitlick, 1987; modified from Jusko, 1976, with permission).

---

59 Ataxia is a common dose-related side effect of high plasma phenytoin levels

---

Subtle, nonsignificant, abnormalities of smooth pursuit of the eyes may be detected in many patients, even at low phenytoin levels. Above 20 mg/l, nystagmus occurs on lateral gaze and dystaxia may be found on neurologic exam. Above 30 mg/l, obvious gait ataxia is often present. Above 40 mg/l, spontaneous nystagmus – as well as more profound disorders of eye movements – and lethargy may occur (Figure 59.1) (Kutt *et al.*, 1964). However, the range of phenytoin blood levels at which patients experience drug toxicity is very broad. Some may have clinically significant ataxia at a level of 20, while others appear unaffected at 40. Nystagmus on far lateral gaze (usually not clinically significant) may occur with levels in the 10–15 mg/l range (Stensrud and Palmer, 1964; Kutt *et al.*, 1964; Haerer and Grace, 1969).

Buchthal and Svensmark (1959–60) found that acute neurologic side effects such as ataxia and nystagmus did not occur in their patients with levels below 14 mg/l; in the range 15–29 mg/l only 15% complained of toxicity and in the range 30–60 mg/l, 26% had none, 24% mild, and 50% severe toxicity (Buchthal

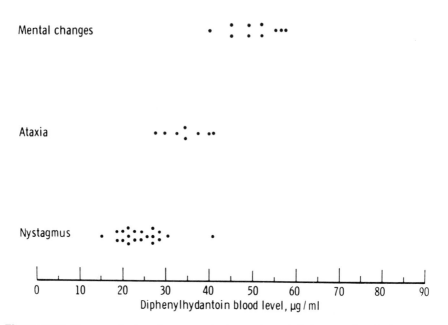

Figure 59.1 The onset of nystagmus, ataxia, and mental changes in relation to phenytoin level (from Kutt *et al.*, 1964).

and Svensmark, 1959–1960; Buchthal *et al.*, 1960). In a study of 110 patients taking PHT, Triedman *et al.* (1960) found that all 19 patients with ataxia or lethargy had blood levels above 30 mg/l, whereas of the 91 nontoxic patients, only 13 had levels above 30 mg/l and 1 was above 50 mg/l. Neurologic side effects were associated with significantly higher PHT levels (13.4 ± 5.5 *vs* 18.4 ± 8.2 mg/l) in a study by Herranz *et al.* (1988).

Discerning an association between specific measures of drug toxicity and blood levels can be difficult, especially within the 'therapeutic' range (Schumacher *et al.*, 1991). A single blood level has poor predictive value for clinical side effects in an individual patient. After several levels are available, however, and after these levels can be correlated with effects in the patient, a good idea of the patient's response pattern can be deduced. The importance of blood levels in evaluating PHT toxicity was underlined by a recent reanalysis of a study which had originally been interpreted as showing that phenytoin had greater adverse neuropsychological adverse effects than did carbamazepine. When patients with high drug levels were eliminated, there was no neuropsychological difference between PHT and CBZ (Dodrill and Troupin, 1991). The neuropsychological effects of antiepileptic drugs are discussed in Principle 98.

Like carbamazepine, phenytoin occasionally causes movement disorders, particularly in patients who have severe secondary generalized epilepsies with underlying neuropathological changes.

The range of free levels at which patients experience toxicity is, as for total levels, very broad (Lesser *et al.*, 1984). Booker and Darcy (1973) reported a closer correlation of drug toxicity with free than with total PHT measurements, but their patients were taking other drugs in addition to PHT, making the study difficult to interpret. In the evaluation of toxicity in a study of outpatients with normal renal function, free PHT showed a slightly better correlation (R = 0.59) than did total PHT (R = 0.49); the toxicity score was determined by a blind rater (Theodore *et al.*, 1985a).

Peripheral neuropathy associated with prolonged phenytoin therapy is usually subclinical, and may be caused by folate deficiency rather than by a direct drug effect (Shorvon and Reynolds, 1982). There is little evidence for permanent cerebellar damage due to phenytoin (Theodore *et al.*, 1987d).

---

60 Some patients on phenytoin get swollen gums

The longer a drug is used, the more that certain side effects become apparent. In the Veterans' Administration Cooperative Study, fewer toxicity-associated dropouts occurred among patients taking phenytoin than any of the other drugs (Mattson *et al.*, 1985). One of the most common systemic complications is gingival hypertrophy, which can affect, in varying degrees, as many as 50% of patients taking the drug (Reynolds, 1989). Although this adverse effect may be less common in patients in the community as a whole than those referred to epilepsy centers (Thomason *et al.*, 1992), there is no increase in alveolar bone loss compared to patients taking carbamazepine (Dahllof *et al.*, 1993). Coarsened facial features and calvarial thickening have also been reported, particularly in patients with severe seizures and underlying neurologic disorders; most of these patients, however, were taking other drugs in addition to phenytoin (Lefebvre *et al.*, 1972). Gum hypertrophy can be reduced by rigorous oral hygiene and usually disappears six months after phenytoin has been discontinued (Dallof *et al.*, 1991; Thomason *et al.*, 1992).

Phenytoin has a number of endocrine side effects, some of which are common to all hepatic enzyme enhancing antiepileptic drugs. The drug reduces T4 binding to thyroxine binding globulin and enhances T4 conversion to T3. TSH should be normal if the patient is clinically euthyroid and is a good screening test. Vitamin D turnover may be increased by phenytoin and calcium absorption may be reduced. Supplementation may be appropriate for patients who have had frequent fractures or who demonstrate osteomalacia (Reynolds, 1989). Phenytoin can impair glucose-stimulated insulin release; a few cases of nonketotic hyperglycemia have been reported (Malherbe *et al.*, 1972). Steroid turnover is increased by the drug and oral contraceptives may be less effective.

Occasionally, patients taking phenytoin develop megaloblastic anemia related to low folate levels which may also lead to reduced vitamin B12 absorption. Hypersensitivity reactions include rashes, lymphadenopathy, and a 'systemic lupus erythematosus' syndrome; these adverse effects usually clear when the drug is stopped (Reynolds, 1989). If clinically significant hepatotoxicity occurs, it usually appears within the first two months of starting the drug and is usually associated with diffuse hypersensitivity.

61 Do not give phenytoin intramuscularly

Phenytoin is soluble only in very alkaline solutions; when injected intramuscularly, it may precipitate and crystalize in the muscle and cause local hemorrhage and necrosis (Serrano and Wilder, 1974). Propylene glycol, the solvent used, may contribute to the toxicity of the drug. Absorption from this depot may be slow and erratic, making difficult the maintenance of therapeutic plasma levels. The drug may continue to be absorbed from the depot long after it was administered and toxicity may occur. Nomograms for intramuscular dosing after oral or intravenous (IV) loading have been developed.

Intramuscular administration can occasionally be useful when patients are unable to take oral phenytoin or are at increased risk for cardiac toxicity from intravenous drug – such as in the elderly. Because of the slow absorption, giving intramuscular phenytoin to a patient in status epilepticus is pointless, even if an IV cannot be started (Principle 83). Although once-a-day administration of intramuscular phenytoin after oral or intravenous loading can be used to maintain therapeutic plasma levels (Wilder and Ramsay, 1976), the large volumes of solution require injections at multiple sites and blood levels must to be monitored frequently. These difficulties seem to vitiate the advantages of being able to give phenytoin intramuscularly. In unconscious patients, phenytoin can often be given via nasogastric tube; alternatively, slow intravenous administration is safe (Principle 83).

62 Phenytoin and carbamazepine can be used together

Phenytoin and carbamazepine are the two most effective drugs for the treatment of complex partial seizures, the most common seizure type in patients with uncontrolled epilepsy (Mattson *et al.*, 1985). These drugs may share a common mechanism of action, the blocking of voltage-dependent sodium channels (Rogawski and Porter, 1990). Experiments in mice detected no advantage of the combination over either drug alone in preventing maximal electroshock seizures, since increased effectiveness was balanced by increased toxicity (Morris *et al.*, 1987). Analysis of brain concentrations suggested an additive rather than synergistic effect, implying that increasing the dose of one of the drugs would be as useful as using the two drugs together.

There is some preliminary human data, however, which suggests that the combination may be useful in patients who have not responded to one or the other drug (Schmidt, 1982; Callaghan *et al.*, 1985; Mattson *et al.*, 1985; Lorenzo *et al.*, 1988). Both drugs are well-tolerated, have low toxicity, and are relatively inexpensive – particularly when compared to the newer antiepileptic drugs. Interactions can be managed by appropriate dose adjustments (Browne *et al.*, 1988).

The combination of carbamazepine and valproic acid has also been reported to improve patients who have not responded to one drug (Dean and Penry, 1988). Other combinations of old and new drugs have not been methodically tested. Seizure treatment is still an empirical enterprise.

---

63 Plasma drug levels should be at the upper end of the therapeutic range in patients with refractory epilepsy

Many authors have noted that some patients tolerate blood levels of carbamazepine and phenytoin that are much higher than the suggested 'therapeutic range' (Buchthal and Svensmark, 1959–60; Kutt *et al.*, 1975; Monaco *et al.*, 1976; Simonsen *et al.*, 1976; Troupin *et al.*, 1977). Others have observed that patients with severe epilepsy may need high blood levels for seizure control (Schmidt, 1983). Lesser *et al.* (1984), for example, reported that 15 of 25 patients (previously treated with multiple drugs) had a 65–100% reduction in seizure frequency when mean plasma carbamazepine concentrations were increased to 11 mg/l, and phenytoin concentrations were increased to 29.4 mg/l. Adverse drug effects were mild. A case report is instructive:

A 20-year-old man had the onset of generalized tonic–clonic seizures at the age of 8 years, followed by complex partial seizures at the age of 9 years. The latter were characterized by a simple partial onset, with 'ringing in the ears', followed by staring, drooling, and loss of consciousness for 2 minutes, followed by a gradual return to normal consciousness over 3 to 5 minutes. Tiredness followed each attack. By age 16 years, the patient was having monthly seizures, and his behavior at home was nearly intolerable; it was clearly worsened by barbiturates. A regimen of phenytoin and carbamazepine was started. Although these two drugs had previously been tried, the maximally tolerated dose of phenytoin had been 300 mg/day, and carbamazepine 800 mg/day. Over many months, the barbiturate was discontinued, and phenytoin and carbamazepine were increased, using a four-times-a-day regimen (similar to that described in Principle 63). Each drug was pushed to maximally tolerated doses, with occasional temporary toxicity from each. Diplopia was the presenting sign of toxicity for each drug, and plasma drug levels were measured to determine which drug was the toxic offender. Eventually, the patient was able to tolerate 425 mg/day of phenytoin and 1,100 mg/day of carbamazepine. From morning blood samples, plasma levels of phenytoin remained in the range of 17–20 μg/ml, and plasma levels of carbamazepine in the range of 6.5–7.5 μg/ml.

On this regimen, the patient's behavior improved dramatically, and his seizures decreased from one a month to one every 6 months. He graduated from high school and college and he has been fully employed for several years.

The major adverse effects of phenytoin and carbamazepine – double vision, nystagmus, dystaxia – are easily evaluated by neurologic examination; further, the effect of these drugs can be tracked relatively easily and safely beyond the 'therapeutic range'. Sedative–hypnotic agents such as phenobarbital present a different problem; patients may appear to become tolerant to the initial drowsiness, but in fact may suffer progressive subtle impairment of higher cognitive function (Mattson and Cramer, 1989). A significant inverse relationship exists between phenobarbital levels and neuropsychological performance (Painter, 1989; Meador et al., 1990). Patients on high doses of barbiturates should be questioned carefully concerning intellectual performance.

The new antiepileptic drugs present yet another difficulty, since their therapeutic ranges are not established and the maximal tolerated doses almost certainly have not been used in clinical trials (Chapter 11). In the 'pre-antiepileptic drug level era', it was standard practice to increase drug doses until clinical toxicity was observed, after which the dose was reduced slightly (Yahr et al., 1952). Until more data are available, this approach should be used when the new drugs are tried – rather than restricting doses to an artificial ceiling.

PRINCIPLE 63

11 Therapy: New and Experimental Drugs

---

64 Felbamate may be useful for the Lennox–Gastaut syndrome as well as for partial seizures, but should be used cautiously due to the risk of aplastic anemia

---

Felbamate (Felbatol) was the first drug for epilepsy to be approved in the United States for 15 years, although several others have already or will soon follow. Although felbamate has a structure similar to the antianxiety drug meprobamate, it does not share the clinical effects of the latter. In animal tests, felbamate is effective against both maximal electroshock and pentylenetetrazole-induced seizures, suggesting that it may be useful for generalized as well as partial seizure disorders (Rogawski and Porter, 1990). The mechanism of action is unknown, but some evidence suggests that it may interact with both gamma-aminobutyric acid (GABA)-benzodiazepine and excitatory amino acid receptors (Rho *et al.*, 1994).

Felbamate has been studied in several clinical trials of complex partial seizures (CPS). Theodore *et al.* (1991) used a three-period crossover design (to estimate the importance of carryover effects) at a single center with 28 patients; these patients were required to have at least 2 CPS per week on carbamazepine (CBZ). Seizure frequency was 14% lower on FBM. Mean FBM levels were 39 ± 11.5 mg/l and CBZ levels decreased by 24%. Leppik *et al.* (1991) reported a two-center study of 56 patients taking PHT and CBZ; their patients were required to have at least 4 seizures per month. Seizure frequency was 7.6% lower on FBM than during baseline and 17.5% lower than on placebo. The mean FBM level was 32.5 mg/l. CBZ levels decreased by 19%. Both of these studies probably used suboptimal FBM doses – only 2300–3000 mg/day.

Two studies compared FBM at 3600 mg/day (mean level 60–80 mg/l) to 15 mg/kg/day of valproate in a total of 155 patients. The patients were required to have at least 8 partial seizures during a 56 day baseline (Sachdeo *et al.*, 1992; Faught *et al.*, 1993), and their other AEDs were discontinued by study day 28. During the 112 day trial, patients on valproate were significantly more likely to drop out from increased seizure frequency or severity. In a multi-center study of 64 patients who were being monitored for possible surgery, the time to fourth seizure was significantly longer on 3600 mg/day (mean level 65.1) with FBM than with placebo (Bourgeois *et al.*, 1993). In this study, patients were maintained on therapeutic levels of at least one other drug; fluctuations in the levels of these drugs were not reported.

FBM is especially unusual – among both the new and the old AEDs – in its potential effectiveness for the Lennox–Gastaut syndrome. Seventy-three patients, each taking up to two antiepileptic drugs (ages 4–36, mean 13) with (a) at least 90 atonic or atypical absence seizures per month, (b) slow spike-wave on EEG, and (c) no evidence of progressive neurological disease, were treated for 70 days with either FBM (45 mg/kg or 3600 mg/day) or placebo (Felbamate Study Group in Lennox–Gastaut syndrome, 1993). FBM reduced all seizures by 19% – and specifically atonic seizures by 34%. The effect appeared to be greater at 45 mg/kg/day (mean level 43.8 mg/l) than at 15 mg/kg/day.

Preliminary reports suggest that FBM may also be effective in other seizure types such as absence (Devinsky *et al.*, 1992) or juvenile myoclonic epilepsy (Sachdeo *et al.*, 1992) when other drugs have failed. Although these results are consistent with the effect found in Lennox–Gastaut syndrome, they have not yet been confirmed by controlled studies.

Felbamate has significant drug interactions; it increases PHT and valproic acid (VPA) levels while lowering CBZ levels by about 20% (Palmer and McTavish 1993). In spite of the decreases in carbamazepine levels, the CBZ epoxide is increased and the overall therapeutic effect may not be changed; the lower CBZ levels did, however, appear to be important in one study (Theodore *et al.*, 1991). Felbamate levels are lowered by hepatic enzyme-inducing drugs such as CBZ and PHT (Palmer and McTavish, 1993).

Felbamate's major adverse effects are GI distress, weight loss, headache, and insomnia (Theodore *et al.*, 1991; Leppik *et al.*, 1991; Sachdeo *et al.*, 1992, Bourgeois *et al.*, 1993; Faught *et al.*, 1993). Diplopia, blurred vision, and ataxia have been reported in add-on trials, but may have been caused in part by fluctuations in other AED levels.

Felbamate has been reported to be associated with aplastic anemia. Twenty-two cases, including three fatalities – two of them children, aged 6 and 14 years, had been reported to the manufacturer as of August 1994 (Wallace Laboratories, personal communication). These patients had been taking felbamate for 2–8 months before their blood dyscrasia was detected. Only two were on mono-therapy; one had discontinued felbamate, and had been taking valproic acid and lamotrigine for several months before aplastic anemia was detected. A single case of thrombocytopenia has been reported (Ney *et al.*, 1994). A number of hepatic fatalities have also occurred in patients taking felbamate.

Approximately 100,000 patients have received felbamate, but many for less than a year. It will be difficult to estimate the true risk of hematologic complications until more data are available. It seems prudent to use felbamate only if there are no alternatives, or in patients already on the drug whose clinical response warrants continued exposure. Although early detection of aplastic anemia may not change the clinical course, patients taking felbamate should have CBCs every 2–4 weeks, at least for the first year of therapy.

A starting dose of 1200 mg/day is reasonable, with increases of 600 mg/week. Although 3600 mg/day has been approved, the maximum dose will probably be in the range of 4000–5000 mg. Patients taking FBM alone will need lower doses to achieve a therapeutic effect. On the other hand, adverse effects in clinical trials have been more frequent when FBM is given with other drugs. Even though felbamate has a half-life of 12–20 hours, three or four doses per day may be required to reduce GI side effects. Based on very limited data, the therapeutic range may be 50–100 mg/l (Theodore *et al.*, 1994a). The maximum recommended dose for children is 45 mg/kg.

---

65 Gabapentin has no significant drug interactions

Gabapentin, although structurally related to GABA, does not appear to act via the GABA system, but binds to a novel brain receptor of unknown function (Porter and Rogawski, 1993). It is active in both maximal electroshock and pentylenetetrazol models, although it is less potent in the latter than is felbamate (Rogawski and Porter, 1990). The drug has recently been approved for adjunctive use in patients with partial seizures. A number of controlled trials in patients with partial seizures have been reported.

In a 12-week multi-center US trial of 306 patients, the median seizure frequency reduction was 24% at 600 mg/day, 20% at 1200, and 32% at 1800 (US Gabapentin Study Group, 1993). Similar results were found in European trials of an additional 500 patients (Leiderman, 1993). Overall, 20–30% of patients had a seizure reduction of at least 50%. There is some evidence for a better response at 1800 than 1200 mg/day; even higher doses (>3000 mg/day) are well tolerated. For this reason, the effect of gabapentin was likely underestimated in these studies. Clinical trials in other epilepsy syndromes are underway.

Since gabapentin is not metabolized by the liver, not bound to plasma proteins, and eliminated unchanged by the kidneys, it does not interact with other drugs. The dose might have to be reduced in patients with renal failure (Bialer, 1993). Sleepiness, dizziness, and ataxia are the major adverse effects; sleepiness occurred in 20% of patients on gabapentin compared to 10% on placebo (US Gabapentin Study Group, 1993; Leiderman, 1993). Although the half-life is only 5–7 hours, there is evidence for a longer pharmacodynamic effect. Brain levels are 80% of plasma levels, but guidelines for gabapentin blood level monitoring have not been established (Foot and Wallace, 1991; Leiderman, 1993).

Because of the short half-life of gabapentin, the drug should be given in three divided doses – at least until more evidence for a longer pharmacodynamic effect appears. The drug can be titrated rapidly, increasing by 300 mg/day to an initial target dose of 1800 (Ramsay, 1994). Faster dose increases can be undertaken cautiously if clinically indicated; in some clinical trials, titration up to 3600 mg over three days has been achieved. Although the maximum tolerated dose is unknown, absorption of the drug decreases above 3600 mg/day.

66 Lamotrigine is effective against partial seizures

Lamotrigine (LTG) was developed as an antifolate agent, but its effect against seizures appears to be unrelated to folic acid metabolism; its mechanism of action is unknown (Rogawski and Porter, 1990; Porter and Rogawski, 1993). Like phenytoin and carbamazepine, it is active in the maximal electroshock but not the pentylenetetrazole model.

LTG trials have probably used suboptimal doses. At 200 mg/day, a 17% decrease in seizures was found; side effects were not significantly different from placebo (Binnie et al., 1989). In a study of 216 patients with partial seizures, seizure frequency decreased by 8% on placebo, 20% on 300 mg/day LTG, and 36% on 500 mg/day (Matsuo et al., 1993). One-third of the patients on 500 mg/day had a 50% or greater decrease in seizures. One study reported that health-related quality of life assessments showed a greater positive effect from LTG than would be predicted by seizure reduction alone, perhaps because of reduced toxicity compared to the other drugs these patients had been taking previously (Smith et al., 1993). In long-term studies, doses up to 700 mg/day are well-tolerated (Pellock et al., 1993).

Both the maximum tolerated dose and the effective blood levels are unknown. At 400 mg/day, the mean steady state level was 2.9 ± 1.3 mg/l (Messenheimer et al., 1994). The drug should probably be started at 100 mg/day, and increased by 100 mg/week. The most common adverse effects have been headache, sleepiness, dizziness, double vision, and ataxia (Matsuo et al., 1993; Pellock et al., 1993). About 2–3% of patients had to stop the drug because of rash. Lamotrigine has a half-life of 25 hours – which is reduced to 15 hours by enzyme inducers like PHT or CBZ, but which is increased to 60 hours by valproate (Ramsay, 1993a). The drug does not affect the metabolism of other AEDs.

67 Vigabatrin has a definite mechanism of action

Vigabatrin is unusual among AEDs in that it appears to do exactly what it was designed to do – irreversibly inhibit the GABA degradative enzyme, GABA transaminase, thereby increasing brain and CSF GABA levels (Ben-Menachem *et al.*, 1988). In European double-blind, placebo-controlled trials of adults at doses of 2–3 g/day, the number of patients with partial seizures reporting a 50% or greater seizure frequency reduction ranged from 30–60%; in smaller groups of patients, thought to have primary generalized epilepsy, 40% had a similar response (Reynolds, 1992). Browne *et al.* (1987) reported a mean decrease in seizures from 11 to 5 per month on 50 mg/kg (maximum 4 g/day). In one study, some patients appeared to have more frequent seizures when the dose was increased from two to three g/day (McKee *et al.*, 1993).

Several preliminary studies have suggested that vigabatrin may be effective in children with infantile spasms or the Lennox–Gastaut syndrome (Gram *et al.*, 1992). The effect may be greater in patients with tuberous sclerosis, some of whom had complete seizure control for long follow-up periods.

Since vigabatrin has been used in Europe for several years, considerable long-term data is available. Patients seen at an epilepsy center were less likely to continue on the drug for more than 6 months than those evaluated at a general neurology clinic (30% *vs* 40%) – perhaps because the former had more severe seizure disorders or perhaps because of alternative therapies such as surgery (Sander *et al.*, 1990).

Vigabatrin has few significant drug interactions and predominantly renal excretion. Several studies reported a decrease in PHT levels of 20%, which may be related to changes in compliance (Browne *et al.*, 1987; Rey *et al.*, 1992). The most prominent side effects are related to CNS depression; sleepiness was reported by 27% of patients on vigabatrin, compared to 13% on placebo (Reynolds, 1992). Psychosis has been attributed to vigabatrin therapy in up to 7% in some series (Sander *et al.*, 1991; Reynolds, 1992). High vigabatrin doses caused intramyelinic edema and CNS vacuolization in rodents and dogs, but evidence for a similar phenomenon in humans has not been found in evoked potential studies, in imaging studies, or in autopsy and neurosurgical specimens (Hammond *et al.*, 1992).

Vigabatrin half-life is only 5–7 hours. The onset of clinical effect is delayed, and probably lasts longer than drug presence in plasma (Rey *et al.*, 1992). The drug can be started at 1 g/day (for adults) and titrated over 3–4 weeks to a maximum of 3000–4000 mg/day. Patients with a history of psychiatric illness should be given vigabatrin with extreme caution. Doses of 40–80 mg/kg/day have been used in children.

68 The choice among the new antiepileptic drugs for partial seizures may depend mainly on pharmacology and side effects

Felbamate, gabapentin, lamotrigine, and vigabatrin have all been effective in clinical trials of patients with uncontrolled partial and secondarily generalized seizures. The role of these new drugs in epilepsy therapy will emerge over time. At the very least, these drugs are worth trying in patients with partial seizures who have not responded to, or cannot tolerate, PHT or CBZ. The choice among them will probably be based on differences in side effects.

Detailed comparisons are difficult because of differences in study methodology and differences in the way in which the study results have been analyzed and reported. Nevertheless, the efficacy of the four drugs appears to be similar. Mean seizure frequency reduction is usually about 30%; occasional patients may have a better response – or, rarely, become seizure-free – even if they have not responded to other drugs such as carbamazepine, phenytoin, or valproic acid. Since most of the patients given these drugs in clinical trials had seizures which were refractory to CBZ and PHT, the effect in patients with less severe epilepsy may be greater. Felbamate and perhaps vigabatrin maybe useful in children with either the Lennox–Gastaut syndrome or infantile spasms; use of the other agents in these syndromes has not yet been reported.

There is no evidence that any of the new drugs is superior to CBZ or PHT for treating CPS or GTCS in non-refractory patients. However, some people may respond better, or have less toxicity, from one drug than another. Felbamate has been approved for monotherapy, but there is no clinical reason why the other new drugs cannot also be tried alone. In combination, gabapentin and vigabatrin are the easiest to use from a pharmacologic point of view because of their limited drug interactions. Plasma levels may be of limited value for these two drugs. Felbamate should be utilized like CBZ or PHT; levels of other AEDs have to be monitored when felbamate is given in combination. Felbamate and lamotrigine plasma levels should become generally available in the near future and should be of clinical assistance.

Felbamate appears to differ from the other three new drugs in that its side effects may prove to be related to CNS excitation rather than depression. Clinically, however, its limiting side effect has been gastrointestinal discomfort. Patients may show a clear preference for one set of side effects over another; this preference can be used to guide the choice of new drug. Although the safety profile of all four drugs in animal studies and clinical trials has been good – and apparent teratogenicity risk low – one must remember that patient exposure is still limited compared to older drugs. The true incidence of serious idiosyncratic side effects or teratogenicity is still unknown.

PRINCIPLE 68

Table 68.1 Pharmacokinetics of new antiepileptic drugs

Drug	Half-life (hours)	Metabolism	Protein binding	Plasma levels (mg/l)*
Felbamate	13–23	hepatic	25–30%	20–80
Gabapentin	5–7	70–100% renal	<10%	1–8
Lamotrigine	25	hepatic	55%	0.5–5.0
Vigabatrin	5–7	60–70% renal	<10%	1–50

*Reported in clinical trials: significance uncertain.

---

69 Several additional drugs are undergoing experimental trials

---

Clinical trials continue on a number of other AEDs, especially for partial seizures. These drugs offer an alternative to patients who have not responded to established agents (which now includes a much wider choice), or are not surgical candidates.

Tiagabine is a potent blocker of presynaptic GABA reuptake; the drug is undergoing clinical trials in the USA and Europe (Rogawski and Porter, 1990). It appears to be effective against partial seizures, but adverse effects related to CNS depression may limit its use. Since metabolism is increased by hepatic enzyme-inducing drugs, higher doses can be tolerated in combination therapy.

Topiramate, like CBZ and PHT, is effective in the maximal electroshock (MES) but not the pentylenetetrazol (PTZ) seizure model (Rogawski and Porter, 1990). It has few drug interactions, and appears to be effective in clinical trials of partial seizures.

Flunarizine is a calcium channel blocker which has been marketed for migraine in several countries. Several clinical trials for partial seizures are nearing completion. One interesting feature of the drug is its half-life of 22 days, helpful for compliance, but a disadvantage if adverse effects occur (Binnie, 1989).

Fosphenytoin is a phenytoin prodrug which, unlike phenytoin, is soluble in physiologic solutions; it is rapidly converted to PHT *in vivo*. Studied in clinical trials of status epilepticus, it appears to have fewer cardiac side effects than PHT on intravenous administration and to be equally effective (LeGarda *et al.*, 1993). Several other soluble phenytoin prodrugs are under development.

Several additional drugs are in clinical trials or are approved outside the USA. Clobazam is a 1,5 benzodiazepine which is effective against CPS (Koepppen *et al.*, 1987). Marketed widely outside the USA, claims of reduced neuropsychological toxicity compared to 1,4 substituted compounds like clonazepam have not been confirmed by formal trials (Shorvon, 1989). Clobazam does not affect the metabolism of carbamazepine, phenytoin, phenobarbital or valproic acid. However, carbamazepine, phenytoin, and phenobarbital increase clobazam conversion to N-desmethylclobazam, an active metabolite with a long half-life; these drugs may enhance the sedative effect of clobazam (Sennoune *et al.*, 1992). As with other benzodiazepines, tolerance to its therapeutic effect develops over several months.

Oxcarbazepine is a keto derivative of carbamazepine which rapidly is converted to 10,11-dihydro-10 hydroxycarbamazepine, an active metabolite which appears to be responsible for the drug's therapeutic effect (Dam *et al.*, 1989). Oxcarbazepine does not lead to significant hepatic enzyme induction, which is an advantage for patients taking several drugs (Grant and Faulds, 1992). Efficacy is similar to CBZ, and some investigators have suggested that adverse effects may be less frequent than with carbamazepine (Dam *et al.*, 1989; Friis *et al.*, 1993). Patients with CBZ-induced rashes have been able to tolerate oxcarbazepine.

Zonisamide is a benzisoxasole derivative which shares some of the characteristics of PHT but may interact with the GABA-benzodiazepine receptor complex at therapeutic levels (Rogawski and Porter, 1990). It is effective against partial seizures as well as some varieties of myoclonic epilepsy (Henry *et al.*, 1988; Schmidt *et al.*, 1993). An increased incidence of kidney stones has been reported; the drug is marketed in Japan.

Controlled-release formulations for carbamazepine and valproic acid are under development (Bialer, 1992). Fluctuations in CBZ levels on twice-daily controlled release carbamazepine were significantly lower than on conventional drug and were similar to those observed when patients were taking ordinary, immediate release, carbamazepine four times a day (McKee *et al.*, 1991). Several other extended release formulations have been made, some of which unfortunately result in differences in carbamazepine bioavailability (Reunanen *et al.*, 1992).

---

70 **Vagal nerve stimulation is an alternative experimental treatment**

In some animal studies, vagal nerve stimulation leads to EEG desynchronization and may reduce seizure frequency. Limited human trials have been conducted. Uthman *et al.* (1993) treated 14 patients with refractory partial seizures using a single-blind protocol. During the placebo phase, patients were told that the device was turned on, but no stimuli were delivered. Overall seizure frequency decreased by 46% in the treated group. One of the difficulties in evaluating vagal stimulation is the ability of patients to perceive the stimulus, making a blinded trial difficult to perform. Other possible approaches to controlling the studies include attempting to demonstrate a dose-response curve and assessing for an increasing effect over time (Uthman *et al.*, 1993).

Vagal stimulation is generally well-tolerated, although the device must be implanted surgically. Hoarseness and cough may occur during the stimulus pulses (Uthman *et al.*, 1993).

Previous neurophysiologic approaches to seizure treatment have included cerebellar stimulation and biofeedback. After a fairly long period of intermittent use, Van Buren *et al.* (1978) performed a controlled trial which showed that cerebellar stimulation was ineffective.

12 Therapy: Generalized Seizures

> **71** Use carbamazepine, phenytoin or valproate for generalized tonic–clonic seizures

Several studies have shown that carbamazepine, phenytoin, and valproic acid provide equivalent control of generalized tonic–clonic seizures and that barbiturates are also effective. In the Veterans Administration Cooperative Study, for example, no difference was found among carbamazepine, phenytoin, phenobarbital, and primidone in the control of generalized seizures, although toxicity was greater with the latter two (Mattson *et al.*, 1985).

Valproic acid is less protective than carbamazepine or phenytoin in the rodent maximal electroshock model, which predicts drug effect against human localization-related epilepsy (Rogawski and Porter, 1990). Furthermore, no differences have been found in several comparisons of the effect of carbamazepine or phenytoin or valproic acid on generalized tonic–clonic seizures, although carbamazepine may be less toxic (Ramsay *et al.*, 1983; Wilder *et al.*, 1983; Mattson *et al.*, 1992).

Wilder *et al.* (1983) compared phenytoin (mean trough level 12.6 mg/l) and valproic acid (mean level 57) in patients with an average of 4 seizures per month; 76% of patients randomized to the former and 82% to the latter had no seizures over six months, although, interestingly, 4 of 34 on valproate developed complex partial seizures. Similar results were obtained by Turnbull *et al.* (1982).

Several of the new antiepileptic drugs may also be effective against generalized tonic–clonic seizures, although most of the studies have been designed to evaluate for control of complex partial seizures. Without video-EEG monitoring, distinguishing primary from secondary generalized seizures in clinical trials may be difficult.

Generalized tonic–clonic seizures appear to be easier to control than complex partial seizures (Callaghan *et al.*, 1985; Mattson *et al.*, 1985, 1992). Schmidt *et al.* (1986), for example, found that higher drug levels are needed to control partial than generalized seizures. Complete control of the latter occurred at phenytoin levels of 14 mg/l but the former at 23 mg/l. In patients being withdrawn from phenobarbital, complex partial seizures occur in the 15–20 mg/l range, while generalized tonic–clonic seizures do not show an increase until levels fall considerably lower (Theodore *et al.*, 1987b). Clinically, many patients with localization-related epilepsy, particularly of temporal lobe origin, continue to have frequent complex partial seizures while their generalized tonic–clonic seizures remain well-controlled.

72 The response to antiabsence medication can be quantified

Absence seizures are almost always accompanied by generalized high voltage EEG discharges (with frontal predominance) at 2.5–3.5/second. Even though clinical seizures may not be detected by observers during short bursts, cognitive performance is still decreased. Studies by Porter *et al.* (1973), and Browne *et al.* (1974), showed impaired reaction time in relation to spike-wave discharges (Figures 72.1, 72.2). In effect, every generalized spike-wave discharge represents

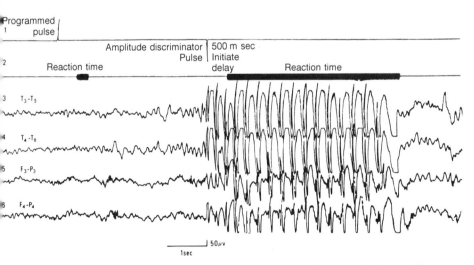

Figure 72.1 Recording from a six-channel polygraph showing reaction time with a 0.5-second delay from the time of onset of generalized spike-and-wave discharge to the time of auditory stimulus. The amplitude discriminator (threshold detector) monitored channel 4 and triggered the stimulus when the EEG amplitude exceeded 100 μV. In this case, the patient responded with a normal reaction time 3 seconds before the paroxysm, but was unable to respond after the paroxysm began; unresponsiveness persisted until the paroxysm ended (from Browne *et al.*, 1974, with permission).

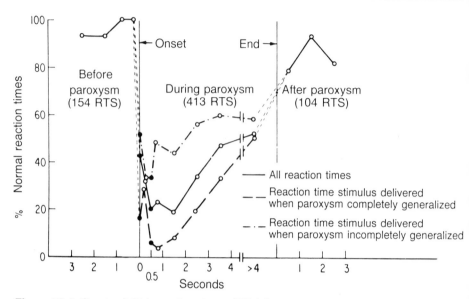

Figure 72.2 Graph of 671 reaction times (RTs) from 26 patients showing percentages of normal reaction times before, during, and after spike-and-wave paroxysms. Patients were least responsive when the paroxysms were completely generalized. There is no evidence of a decrement in consciousness before the onset of the paroxysms, and patients are normally responsive only 2 seconds after the end of the attack (from Browne *et al.*, 1974, with permission).

a short seizure. Even if discharges are not fully generalized, they are still usually associated with impaired cognitive performance (Browne *et al.*, 1974).

EEG monitoring is much more important in patients with absence than other seizure types. In patients with complex partial or secondary generalized seizures, for example, changes in the EEG do not necessarily parallel a patient's clinical course (Theodore *et al.*, 1984c). In absence epilepsy, however, the EEG is a much more reliable measure of seizure frequency and drug effect than is clinical observation, either by trained observers or a patient's family (Browne *et al.*, 1983). If EEGs are not performed, seizure frequency may be underestimated. This is particularly important after treatment is started, since a child thought to be seizure-free may still be having short absence attacks which may impair performance. On occasion, parents and teachers may also overestimate absence frequency.

During treatment, EEGs, should be obtained to check on the effect of drug therapy. These recordings should preferably be longer than routinely performed, as routine tracings have proven to miss a significant number of attacks compared to 12-hour recordings (Browne *et al.*, 1983). The aim of treatment should be to eliminate all abnormal generalized EEG discharges.

PRINCIPLE 72

---

73 Ethosuximide is the treatment of choice for absence seizures that occur alone

About 60–80% of patients can achieve complete seizure control on ethosuximide or valproic acid alone. Ethosuximide is usually chosen first as it is considered to be less toxic, even though short-term formal comparisons have shown little or no difference in efficacy and side effects between the two drugs (Sato et al., 1982). Ethosuximide has a long-half life – more than 30 hours – and can be given once a day, although divided doses may be necessary to reduce gastrointestinal discomfort. Protein binding is less than 10% (Chang, 1989). Ethosuximide does not interact to any clinically significant degree with other antiepileptic drugs. Although there is a clear dose-blood level relationship, it varies dramatically from patient to patient (Sherwin et al., 1973; Browne et al., 1975).

The therapeutic range is 50–100 mg/l, although patients are more likely to become seizure-free at the higher end of the range; the use of plasma levels can dramatically increase the effectiveness of the drug (Figure 73.1). Usually, the drug is started at about 10 mg/kg/day, and increased about every five days to 30–40 mg/kg/day. Children metabolize ethosuximide more quickly than adults and need proportionately higher doses.

Since ethosuximide shows little or no dose-related impairment of cognitive function, high doses may be used in an attempt to control absence seizures completely (Browne et al., 1975). Even a few absences occurring each day during school can disrupt a child's performance. Some patients have been maintained on doses above 70 mg/kg (up to 2000 mg/day) and blood levels above 120 mg/l (Sherwin et al., 1973; Blomquist and Zetterlund, 1985). Patients with normal intelligence and a normal neurologic exam have a better prognosis (Sato et al., 1983).

Gastrointestinal discomfort, including nausea and anorexia, is the most common side effect of ethosuximide (Dreifuss, 1989). Some patients complain of drowsiness at the beginning of treatment. There have been rare reports of behavioral disturbances or acute psychoses, and abnormal involuntary movements, perhaps related to high blood levels, although data are sparse. Skin rashes, and a hypersensitivity syndrome which includes drug-induced systemic lupus erythematosus, have been reported, as well as aplastic anemia and pancytopenia. Because of the age range of patients usually treated with ethosuximide, little data on teratogenicity are available.

Since ethosuximide is useful only for absence seizures, proper differential diagnosis is very important. The physician should also keep in mind that a patient who is initially given a mistaken diagnosis of complex partial seizures and who is already on several drugs which are ineffective for absence seizures will not respond to a 'tentative' low-dose addition of ethosuximide. The other drugs

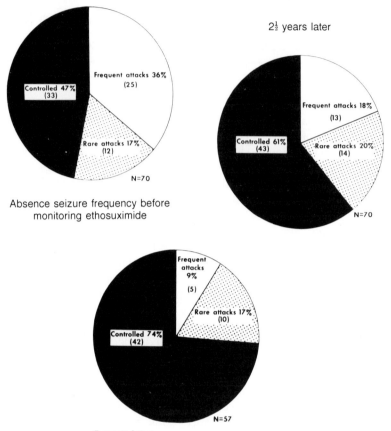

Figure 73.1 The control of absence attacks before monitoring plasma drug levels and 2.5 and 5 years after commencing monitoring. The improvements are highly significant and greatly in excess of what might have been expected from the natural course of remission of absence attacks. Nineteen patients of the original 70 had significant increases in plasma ethosuximide levels after 2.5 years; 13 of these had improved seizure control, including 10 who became seizure-free (from Sherwin, 1982, with permission).

should be tapered to reduce cumulative toxicity and a vigorous trial of ethosuximide initiated.

74 Valproic acid should be used for absence seizures complicated by generalized tonic–clonic seizures

Generalized tonic–clonic seizures may occur in as many as 45% of patients with absence attacks (Loiseau *et al.*, 1983). The generalized tonic–clonic seizures can be present at seizure onset or can begin as long as 16 years after the absence seizures. In most cases they begin earlier; 70–75% will appear by the age of 15 (Dieterich *et al.*, 1985a, 1985b). Some patients whose absence attacks have disappeared completely may subsequently develop generalized tonic–clonic seizures (Currier *et al.*, 1963). However, patients who do develop generalized tonic–clonic seizures are less likely either to achieve full remission of their absence attacks or to have normal intelligence (Sato *et al.*, 1983; Dieterich *et al.*, 1985b).

Ethosuximide is ineffective against generalized tonic–clonic seizures (or indeed any seizure type other than primary generalized absence). Valproic acid, however, is an excellent choice for both seizure types.

In the USA, valproic acid is available as a syrup or capsules. Divalproex is a partially neutralized formulation which is less irritating to the gastrointestinal tract and is now used more frequently than the original formulation. It is also available in 'sprinkles' which have a slower rate of absorption and provide more constant plasma levels. No parenteral form is available, but the syrup is well-absorbed and tolerated when given as an enema diluted with tapwater (Cloyd and Kriel, 1981). Worldwide, other forms are also available (Figure 74.1).

Valproic acid is usually started at about 10 mg/kg/day, and should be gradually increased until absence attacks are controlled. Although many patients can be controlled using 30–60 mg/day, up to 120 mg/day has been used (Covanis *et al.*, 1982; Rowan *et al.*, 1979). Most studies have found a consistent therapeutic valproate effect against primary generalized absence seizures when trough levels

Forms of valproate

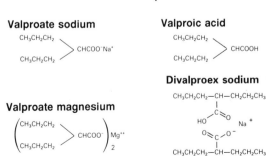

Figure 74.1 Four of the most common forms of valproate (see text).

are in the 50–100 mg/l range; some investigators, however, have reported good results at lower levels (Villareal *et al.*, 1978; Sato *et al.*, 1982; Covanis *et al.*, 1982; Farrell *et al.*, 1986).

Unfortunately, there is wide interindividual variability in the dose–plasma level relationship. In one study, the dose needed to maintain a level of 75 mg/l ranged from 25–150 mg/day (Cloyd *et al.*, 1983). Valproic acid clearance in children is up to three times more rapid than adults; children often need relatively higher doses for therapeutic levels (Dodson and Tasch, 1981; Cloyd *et al.*, 1983). Valproate may have marked fluctuations in serum levels during the course of a day and a single level, even at morning trough, may not provide enough information to make appropriate clinical decisions. Multiple daily dosing is often needed to obtain steady plasma levels.

Probably because of induction of metabolism, higher doses are also needed when valproic acid is given with other drugs (Cloyd *et al.*, 1983). Valproic acid displaces phenytoin from protein binding sites; total levels fall and free levels are either unaffected or rise (Mattson and Cramer, 1989). Valproic acid increases conversion of carbamazepine to carbamazepine epoxide; patients may become toxic despite stable or falling carbamazepine levels unless the metabolite is measured as well (Theodore *et al.*, 1989a). The most important interaction with valproate is inhibition of phenobarbital metabolism; addition of valproate to a patient on phenobarbital may lead to very high barbiturate levels with stupor or coma (Kapetanovic *et al.*, 1981). Valproate may also increase ethosuximide levels (Mattson and Cramer, 1980).

In normal adults, VPA is 87–95% bound to plasma protein; the free fraction increases with increasing plasma levels, and may be twice as high at 100 mg/l as at 50 mg/l (Riva *et al.*, 1983; Bowdle *et al.*, 1980). In patients with renal disease, the unbound fraction may be increased to 20–25% despite normal albumin levels (Gugler and Mueller, 1978). PHT at 20 mg/ml increased the valproate free fraction from 6 to 12% (Cramer and Mattson, 1979). However, measurements of free levels have not provided superior clinical information (Froscher *et al.*, 1985; Barre *et al.*, 1988). Physiologic alterations in plasma lipids may also affect VPA binding.

Valproic acid alone or in combination with ethosuximide is the best treatment for patients experiencing both absence and generalized tonic–clonic seizures. Dieterich *et al.* (1985b) reported that more than 85% of such patients became seizure-free, compared to only 35% who received other drugs.

75 Valproic acid may cause hepatic damage

The most common side effect of valproic acid is gastrointestinal discomfort, which can be alleviated – at least in part – by using divalproex. Some patients tolerate the syrup better than either capsular form. Even though nausea and vomiting are common, appetite is increased and many patients gain weight (Dinesin *et al.*, 1984). Tremor and other neurologic side effects of valproic acid, especially sedation and alteration of consciousness, do appear to be more common at levels over 100 mg/l, although clinical variation is wide (Chadwick, 1985). These adverse effects often respond to a dose reduction. One recent study found that children without any side effects had a mean level of 60.7 ± 17.5 mg/l, while those with drowsiness had a level of 88 ± 36.9 mg/l (Herranz *et al.*, 1988).

Fatal hepatic failure, which may rarely occur after years of therapy, is the most serious complication of valproic acid (Dreifuss, 1989). Liver function tests may not be abnormal before patients become sick with nausea, vomiting, and lethargy. Initial US experience suggested that the risk was 1/7000 in children under the age of two, but as high as 1/500 among those receiving the drug in combination therapy. A pattern of hepatic damage reminiscent of Reye's syndrome has been blamed on increased production of 4-ene metabolites induced by other antiepileptic drugs, but additional metabolic pathways may be important as well (Dreifuss *et al.*, 1989; Siemes *et al.*, 1993). For patients older than two, there was 1 fatality in 12,000 patients with polytherapy but only 1 in 45,000 with monotherapy.

This initial experience led to a change in prescribing patterns and a marked decrease in reports of hepatic toxicity (Dreifuss *et al.*, 1989). For children under three years, valproic acid should not be given in combination with other antiepileptic drugs unless absolutely necessary. The drug should not be given to patients with either a personal history or a family history of liver disease. Patients on valproic acid should generally avoid aspirin, especially in the first 3–6 months of therapy. If any suspicious symptoms develop, particularly after a febrile illness, the drug should be stopped.

Abdominal pain and vomiting may also be the presenting symptoms of acute pancreatitis, which is usually reversible when valproic acid is stopped, but which may be fatal in approximately 10% of cases (Asconape *et al.*, 1993). Like hepatitis, it occurs more frequently in patients on multiple drugs; 70% of cases were in the first year of therapy.

Valproic acid is associated with a number of other systemic side effects, including hair loss and amenorrhea, both of which may remit despite continued therapy (Dreifuss, 1989). Elevated ammonia and decreased carnitine levels have not been related convincingly to clinical toxicity. Up to one-third of patients receiving long-term therapy develop hematologic abnormalities, particularly low platelet counts (May and Sunder, 1993). These are rarely severe enough to require cessation of therapy; platelet counts usually increase when the drug dose is lowered. Hematologic abnormalities may be associated with serologic evidence for systemic lupus erythematosus (Asconape *et al.*, 1994).

PRINCIPLE 75

76 For drug resistant absence seizures, ethosuximide and valproic acid can be used together

For patients who do not become seizure-free on ethosuximide, valproic acid can be tried. A significant proportion of patients who do not respond to one of these drugs will be helped by the other (Sato *et al.*, 1983). Larger doses than usual may have to be given to maintain therapeutic plasma drug levels. In patients who prove resistant to a single medication, the combination is usually well tolerated, although a few will have increased side effects.

Alternative approaches to the treatment of absence seizures include the use of benzodiazepines, which may be effective for a short time. After several months, however, tolerance develops and seizures recur despite increasing doses (Robertson, 1986). The new antiepileptic drug felbamate has been reported to be helpful in a small number of patients (Principle 64).

Proper use of ethosuximide and valproic acid should lead to seizure control in the majority of patients. Dieterich *et al.* (1985a) followed 194 patients with absence epilepsy up to the age of eighteen. Therapy with ethosuximide and/or valproic acid led to seizure control in 95%, compared to only 45% in patients given other drugs. It is important to continue therapy for several years after seizures stop; 30 patients had at least one relapse after seizure control was attained, usually because of drug doses which were omitted.

77 Atonic seizures are resistant to therapy

Patients with secondary generalized epilepsies and atonic seizures have a poor prognosis for neuropsychological functioning (Loiseau *et al.*, 1983; Brorson and Wranne, 1987) and they do not respond well to most AEDs. Many may have significant underlying neurological disease and are included in the spectrum of the Lennox–Gastaut syndrome (Principle 25). These factors are intertwined; impaired function may indicate more severe pathology and frequent seizures may affect performance. Drugs useful for partial seizures, such as phenytoin, carbamazepine, and the barbiturates, are ineffective for atonic seizures. Some patients may have a good initial response to benzodiazepines. However, the usefulness of these drugs is limited by development of tolerance over several months, as well as their sedative side effects (Robertson, 1986). Some 34% of these patients have a previous history of infantile spasms; corticosteroids have been used in atonic seizures, but no controlled data are available to assess the therapeutic effect (Farrell, 1993b).

Valproic acid is occasionally effective. In the most favorable studies, half the patients had a useful clinical response and as many as one-third became seizure-free – at least for a period of time (Jeavons *et al.*, 1977; Covanis *et al.*, 1982; Henriksen and Johannessen, 1982). Problems with seizure classification – as well as varying etiology – complicate the systematic study of these patients. Many investigators feel that valproic acid plasma levels up to 125 mg/l should be maintained.

The new antiepileptic drug felbamate reduced seizure frequency by about 20% in a controlled trial of children with Lennox–Gastaut syndrome (Principle 64). However, felbamate should be used with caution at this time due to reports of an association with aplastic anemia. Initial reports suggest that vigabatrin may be useful in some patients (Principle 67).

When drugs fail, the ketogenic diet can be tried (Kinsman *et al.*, 1992). This approach is usually more successful in younger children, and entails excellent cooperation among the family, dietician, and physician. Sudden reversal of acidosis can precipitate status epilepticus.

One of the neurologist's most important contributions is to determine the nature of other, associated seizure types (either partial or generalized), of which the atonic attacks may, in fact, be only one component. The following case report characterizes this approach:

A 6-year-old girl was well until the age of 5 years, when she had a generalized tonic–clonic seizure at the time of an earache and a temperature of 103°F. Lumbar puncture revealed normal CSF. Following a second generalized tonic–clonic seizure three weeks later, she was started on phenobarbital, which was later changed to mephobarbital because of severe hyperactivity. The generalized tonic–clonic seizures did not recur, but within a month she began having attacks of bilateral clonic twitching of the face and sudden falling; alteration of consciousness was also apparent. These attacks, which would last from 5 to 15 seconds, occurred 10–15 times a day. One atonic attack caused a head injury with brief loss of consciousness. Phenytoin and clonazepam were added without improvement.

A neurologist specializing in epilepsy saw the patient. He added valproate to the regimen and gradually discontinued all other medications. The withdrawal period was associated with some increased seizures, but the plan, executed over six months, was entirely successful. The child became seizure free on valproate alone.

Unhappily, the most severe atonic attacks are much less responsive than those of the fortunate patient described above.

PRINCIPLE 77

78 Some myoclonic seizures respond dramatically to valproate

Myoclonic seizures occur in a variety of clinical contexts, including the progressive myoclonus epilepsies and Lennox–Gastaut syndrome, and may be very difficult to treat. However, patients with juvenile myoclonic epilepsy respond very well to valproic acid; 80–90% of patients achieve seizure control (Asconape and Penry, 1984; Penry *et al.*, 1989). In addition, valproic acid is probably still the best drug for patients with one of the myoclonus epilepsy syndromes (Koskiniemi *et al.*, 1974; Genton *et al.*, 1990).

Juvenile myoclonic epilepsy is likely to persist into adult life, and indefinite treatment usually often necessary (Delgado-Escueta and Enrile-Bacsal, 1984). Generalized tonic–clonic seizures occur in most patients, particularly if drugs are stopped; up to one third may also have absence attacks (Loiseau *et al.*, 1991). Lack of sleep and alcohol may increase myoclonic jerk frequency.

Patients who do not respond to, or cannot tolerate, valproic acid, may benefit from a drug like carbamazepine for the generalized tonic–clonic seizures and acetazolamide for the myoclonic jerks. The new antiepileptic drug felbamate may be helpful, although it may be associated with an increased incidence of aplastic anemia (Principle 64). In severely affected patients, benzodiazepines may be required and may be used in combination with valproate.

Post-anoxic myoclonus is a syndrome which is usually found in patients who have suffered cardiac arrest and may have severe neurologic impairment. Attempts have been made to treat it with the serotonin precursor L-5-hydroxytryptophan (Van Woert and Rosenbaum, 1979). Valproic acid or felbamate may also be tried.

79 Infantile spasms are difficult to treat

Adrenocorticotrophic hormone (ACTH) has been used for infantile spasms since 1958. Few controlled trials have been performed, however, and the optimal dose remains unknown. Snead *et al.* reported that 100% of patients achieved complete remission on a dose of 150 units/m²/day for one week followed by a taper over eight weeks (Snead *et al.*, 1983). However, 18 of 43 patients had recurrent seizures in the ensuing six to seven months. . In another study, doses of 75 units/m² provided initial control in about 75% of the patients (Farwell *et al.*, 1984). Additional courses of ACTH can, of course, also be tried.

PRINCIPLE 79

In addition to the cycle of seizure remission and relapse, ACTH treatment leads to frequent and significant adverse effects – which rarely may be fatal – including hypertension, metabolic disturbances, cardiomyopathy, infection, and cerebral edema (Dulac and Schlumberger, 1993). Oral steroids may be equally effective, but just as toxic (Hrachovy *et al.*, 1983).

Valproic acid is an alternative therapy. In one study, complete seizure control was achieved at a mean plasma level of 113 mg/l in 11 of 22 patients after four weeks and in 20 patients after six months (Siemes *et al.*, 1988). Dulac and Schlumberger (1993) found that a combination of low dose hydrocortisone and valproic acid controlled seizures in 75% of their patients.

Several experimental drugs may be helpful. Nitrazepam, a benzodiazepine available in other countries, but only for investigational use in the USA, was as effective as ACTH in a randomized study (Dreifuss *et al.*, 1986). Clonazepam does not seem to be as useful, and led to serious adverse effects from respiratory complications (Vassella *et al.*, 1973). Vigabatrin provided seizure control in 43% of patients, including 71% with tuberous sclerosis; the study group included an unusually broad age range, i.e., from 2 months to 13 years (Gram *et al.*, 1992).

Even if seizures are controlled, the prognosis for neurological function is poor; as few as 5% of patients may have normal development (Glaze *et al.*, 1988). Since the presence of an underlying disease appears adversely to affect both seizure control and neurologic outcome, the effect of treatment on neuropsychological function needs to be more rigorously evaluated in controlled trials.

---

80 The benefit of treating febrile seizures is uncertain

Febrile seizures are often terrifying events for families as well as children; the attacks disrupt everyday life, engender the expense of emergency room visits, and evoke fears of later epilepsy. Treatment with phenobarbital and perhaps with valproic acid may reduce recurrence of febrile seizures, but unknown is whether the chance of developing epilepsy will be reduced by such therapy, even when a child has adverse risk factors (Rosman *et al.*, 1993). Chronic barbiturate therapy may be associated with cognitive deficits and impaired learning; it is possible that these effects may persist even after treatment is stopped (Farwell *et al.*, 1990). Valproic acid, even though well-tolerated in most cases, can cause a wide range of adverse effects. In addition, any chronic drug treatment entails inconvenience and expense.

Oral or rectal diazepam, administered at the time of fever in children with a history of febrile seizures, reduced recurrence significantly, although patients in the treatment group continued to have seizures, in part because the diazepam was not given during all febrile illnesses (Rosman *et al.*, 1993). Nearly 40% of children had some adverse effects from the diazepam.

In a large proportion of children with 'complex' febrile seizures, the first febrile seizure is itself 'complex'. If, therefore, the seizures are responsible for neurologic damage – such as the development of hippocampal sclerosis – the insult will already have occurred before treatment could have been started (Verity and Golding, 1991; Kuks *et al.*, 1993). There is no definitive evidence that preventing recurrent febrile seizures reduces the risk of later epilepsy (Verity and Golding, 1991). Chronic antiepileptic drug treatment is not appropriate for most children with febrile seizures, and should only be considered when unequivocal risk factors for the development of epilepsy are present. The physician should make certain that the parents are partners in the therapeutic process, particularly if intermittent treatment at the time of fever is prescribed; they should also understand the rationale for either giving or withholding treatment.

13 Therapy: Status Epilepticus

> ## 81 Drug withdrawal is a common cause of status epilepticus

When patients either forget to take their AEDs, or they suddenly stop taking the drugs on their own initiative, serious clinical problems may occur. Status epilepticus has been reported to be associated with sudden AED withdrawal in up to 25% of cases (Aminoff and Simon, 1980). The risk of seizure exacerbation depends on the drug being stopped.

When patients are withdrawn from either phenobarbital (PB) or primidone, complex partial seizures (CPS) increase in frequency as levels fall through the 15–20 mg/l range, while GTCS occur when levels reach 5–10 mg/l (Theodore *et al.*, 1987b). The initial PB level and the rate of fall do not seem to be related to the seizure exacerbation (Theodore *et al.*, 1987b). Phenytoin (PHT) and carbamazepine (CBZ) do not prevent PB withdrawal seizures, perhaps because their mechanisms of action are different and cross tolerance does not occur. In routine clinical practice, PB withdrawal in outpatients at a rate of about 30 mg/month is usually well-tolerated. Achieving therapeutic levels of the replacement drug before beginning PB taper is reasonable, as the risk of status epilepticus may be reduced even though individual seizures are not prevented (Theodore and Porter, 1983a).

Benzodiazepines are also associated with a large risk of withdrawal seizures. Clonazepam, in particular, may lead to severe exacerbation of seizures during drug withdrawal; seizures may be worse when high doses have been given over a prolonged period (Specht *et al.*, 1989). Sugai (1993) reported that patients whose clonazepam dose was lowered by no more than 0.04 mg/kg/week were less likely to have seizure exacerbations.

Tolerance to the antiepileptic effect of CBZ and PHT does not appear to occur. Some studies suggest that cessation of PHT is not associated with withdrawal seizures (Marciani *et al.*, 1985; Bromfield *et al.*, 1989; Duncan *et al.*, 1990). PHT obeys Michaelis–Menton kinetics, and clearance may be prolonged, especially at higher plasma levels, creating a physiologic taper. In some patients, the drug can be tapered rapidly without risk of an increase in seizure frequency *beyond that due to loss of therapeutic effect*; in patients with moderate or severe epilepsy, however, this maneuver should be undertaken with great caution. One study suggests that a valproic acid taper is not associated with withdrawal seizure exacerbation (Duncan *et al.*, 1990). If in doubt, very slow drug removal is the most conservative and reasonable approach.

Seizure exacerbation has been reported to occur in association with CBZ withdrawal in several studies (Marciani *et al.*, 1985; Duncan *et al.*, 1990). Patients who had their carbamazepine withdrawn over four days experienced significantly more generalized tonic–clonic seizures than those whose drug was withdrawn over ten days (Malow *et al.*, 1993). Some patients were not able to tolerate withdrawal because of increased anxiety and depression, even if these symptoms appeared to be mild and even if the seizure frequency did not change (Ketter *et al.*, 1994).

Finally, when discussing drug withdrawal, one must of course note that alcohol withdrawal is one of the most common drug-related causes of status epilepticus, accounting for 10–40% of cases in some patient populations (Alldredge and Lowenstein, 1993).

---

82 Status epilepticus requires urgent therapy

Generalized tonic–clonic status epilepticus is a medical emergency requiring immediate treatment, both supportive and specific. In general, only intravenous antiepileptic drugs should be used. Although the underlying cause is a significant factor, both mortality and morbidity are also related to the length of status (Rowan and Scott, 1970; Aminoff and Simon, 1980; Treiman, 1993).

Frequently, patients present with a history of a cluster of generalized seizures, separated by brief intervals. If the patient is stuporous between the seizures themselves and does not recover to full alertness, he or she should be treated for status. Even if there is recovery for a period between each seizure, the patient still clearly needs additional antiepileptic drugs immediately. Increasing evidence suggests that the adverse effects even of repeated seizures is significant, and that attempts should be made to stop them as soon as possible (Wasterlain *et al.*, 1993). Individual generalized tonic–clonic seizures usually last less than two minutes and should be treated vigorously if they continue longer than that period (Theodore *et al.*, 1994b).

Absence status and complex partial status are less common than generalized tonic–clonic status. They often present diagnostic dilemmas, masquerading as psychiatric disease. Although they should be treated vigorously, intravenous drugs may not be needed.

When a patient presents in generalized tonic–clonic status, adequacy of the airway should be confirmed; intubation may be needed, particularly if the seiz-ures do not respond to initial therapy. Two intravenous lines should be started, one with normal saline for the intravenous phenytoin administration and one for glucose; after drawing blood samples for chemistry, hematology, drug screens (and antiepileptic drug levels if the patient is suspected of taking them), thiamine and glucose can be given. It is very important to take the patient's temperature, since hyperthermia is a serious complication of status. Arterial blood gases can also be obtained.

During status epilepticus patients develop lactic acidosis from intense muscle activity; the problem usually resolves spontaneously. Initial hypertension and hyperglycemia from catecholamine release may be followed by hypotension if the seizures are not controlled (Walton, 1993). Acute rhabdomyolysis and renal failure may occur after prolonged status.

Common causes of status include antiepileptic drug withdrawal, overdoses of other therapeutic drugs such as theophylline, systemic metabolic disorders, and intracranial disease. Barry and Hauser (1993) reported that only 23% of patients with a history of epilepsy, compared to 88% with no history, had an immediately apparent cause for their status. However, patients with a history of seizures may have therapeutic levels of one or more antiepileptic drugs at the time the status begins, suggesting the importance of factors other than drug withdrawal (Barry and Hauser, 1994). Once the patient is stable, MRI scanning can be performed if clinically indicated. Suspicion of infection should lead to a lumbar puncture; status itself can evoke a peripheral leukocytosis as well as a CSF pleocytosis (Aminoff and Simon, 1980).

Treatment for status should proceed in an orderly manner, with careful plan-ning for the next step at each stage of treatment. The physician should alert appropriate support services, such as anesthesiology, that their help may be needed. Specific drug therapy is discussed in Principle 83.

---

83 Intravenous drugs should be used to treat status epilepticus

Rapid onset of action, when combined with maximal bioavailability, is essential for the treatment of status epilepticus. Only intravenous drugs should be used unless venous access is impossible.

In order to obtain rapid seizure control, a benzodiazepine, either 10–20 mg of diazepam or 4–8 mg of lorazepam, should be given first (Leppik *et al.*, 1983; Treiman, 1990; Ramsay, 1993b). The dose can be adjusted for body weight and size. The dose can be repeated after five to ten minutes if seizures are not controlled. Lorazepam has a longer duration of action than diazepam, and seizures are less likely to restart because of falling plasma levels. Initial seizure control can be obtained in 70–80% of patients with this regimen (Treiman, 1990). Respiratory depression is the major complication of benzodiazepines; for any patient in status, assisted ventilation should be available if needed.

If seizures do not stop after the administration of diazepam or lorazepam, intravenous phenytoin should be given, in a dose of 20 mg/kg. Glucose must not be in the intravenous line used for phenytoin administration to avoid crystallization of the drug. The infusion rate, if possible, should be lower than 50 mg/minute – and no more than 25 mg/minute in the elderly – to prevent hypotension and cardiac arrhythmias (Cranford et al., 1979). ECG monitoring is helpful but PHT infusion should be started even if there is a delay in hooking up the EEG equipment; blood pressure should be checked frequently.

In elderly women in particular, intravenous phenytoin (particularly if given at an infusion rate greater than 25 mg/minute and if given through a small bore catheter) may cause soft tissue injury and even, rarely, loss of a limb (Spengler et al., 1988).

Even if benzodiazepines have controlled the seizures, the patient needs to have therapeutic levels of a non-sedative drug so that seizures do not recur and so that mental status can be evaluated. Intravenous phenytoin is often the drug of choice. The risk of inducing drug toxicity from giving a 'loading dose' of phenytoin to a patient who may already be taking the drug is much less than the risk of recurrent status, which may be difficult to stop.

After the administration of benzodiazepines and phenytoin, at least 90% of patients will have cessation of their seizures; many who have not responded will have acute severe CNS disease. Phenobarbital should be given next, to a dose of 20 mg/kg, and at a rate of 50 to 100 mg/minute. At this stage the patient should be in an intensive care unit with both EEG and ECG monitoring; the patient is usually intubated. If phenobarbital does not stop the seizures, coma can be induced with pentobarbital (15 mg/kg, followed by 1.5 mg/kg/hr) or thiopental 4 mg/kg, followed by 1–4 mg/kg/hr). Thiopental is taken up into the brain more rapidly and is metabolized to the longer half-life pentobarbital. The dose of either drug should be large enough to suppress all epileptiform discharges. Phenobarbital is less useful for prolonged barbiturate coma because its long half-life makes the effect take longer to abate when the drug is stopped. Barbiturate coma may cause hypotension requiring pressors (Yaffe and Lowenstein, 1993).

After each drug has been given, the next should be started immediately if seizures do not stop. Although the risk of hemodynamic and respiratory complications increases with cumulative drug administration, these can usually be managed with appropriate supportive care.

In the rare event that intramuscular therapy must be given, midazolam is absorbed more rapidly after intramuscular administration than other benzodiazepines. Phenytoin prodrugs with better intramuscular absorption may become available, but their onset of action will still be very much slower than intravenous phenytoin (Leppik et al., 1990).

PRINCIPLE 83

14 Therapy: The Role of Sedative Antiepileptic Drugs

> ## 84 The role of barbiturates and benzodiazepines should be limited

Any long-term antiepileptic medication – especially at high levels – is subject to scrutiny for its subtle effects on cognition and memory. Non-sedative drugs like phenytoin, for example, have been reported to have deleterious effect on mental function by some investigators (Smith *et al.*, 1987), although other studies have not confirmed these observations (Meador *et al.*, 1993). The evidence indicates, however, that the worst offenders in this regard are the barbiturates and the benzodiazepines, which are still considered by many to be essential for the chronic treatment of epilepsy.

One possible – although somewhat oversimplified – measure of sedative potential of the various antiepileptic drugs may be the presenting dose-related side effect. Not all antiepileptic drugs produce sedation as the first sign of adverse effects. Of the older antiepileptic drugs derived from the heterocyclic ring shown in Figure 84.1, those that retain the 5-membered ring (e.g., phenytoin and ethosuximide) rarely present with sedation as the first adverse effect; phenytoin usually presents with nystagmus, ataxia, and diplopia, and ethosuximide with gastrointestinal distress. Presenting with sedation and sleep, however, are the barbituric acid derivatives, which have a 6-membered ring structure (Porter and Theodore, 1986).

Evidence for the direct deleterious effects of barbiturates on general intelligence, perceptual motor tests, memory, performance tests, and behavior has been reviewed in a study of the removal of sedative–hypnotic antiepileptic drugs (Theodore and Porter, 1983a). In a study by Vining *et al.* (1987), 21 children with epilepsy were given, in a double-blind crossover design, either phenobarbital or valproate. Therapeutic plasma levels of each drug were maintained for six months. Deleterious effects on Wechsler Intelligence Scale results and other performance test scores during phenobarbital administration documented the interference in mental function caused by phenobarbital as compared with a

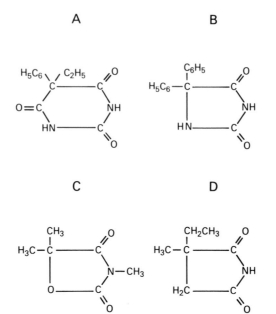

Figure 84.1 The cyclic ureide structure of antiepileptic drugs developed through the late 1950s. (A) phenobarbital; (B) phenytoin; (C) trimethadione; (D) ethosuximide. From Porter (1986).

nonsedative antiepileptic drug. Theodore and Porter (1983a) removed all sedative antiepileptic drugs from 78 patients with severe epilepsy. No patient was left on a barbiturate, desoxybarbiturate, benzodiazepine, or even bromide. The regimens were altered to include only appropriate nonsedative drugs at appropriate doses. Seizure frequency actually improved in some patients, and only one patient was worse. Toxicity was decreased in 46 patients (59%), with decreases noted in diplopia, ataxia, daytime sleepiness, and behavior problems. This study shows that sedative antiepileptic drugs are not necessary for optimal seizure control, even in severely affected patients, and that the removal of such drugs from the regimen may decrease medication toxicity.

In one psychometric and behavioral study of children, no differences were found between patients on carbamazepine and phenobarbital (Mitchell and Chavez, 1987). In another study, however, children treated with phenobarbital had a much higher prevalence of major depressive disorders than those treated with carbamazepine (Brent et al., 1987). In patients with febrile seizures treated with phenobarbital, moreover, adverse effects on IQ scores appeared to persist for up to six months after the drug was stopped (Farwell et al., 1990).

Important evidence from metabolic studies such as positron emission tomography (PET) has documented that, even at therapeutic doses and levels, phenobarbital depresses human cerebral glucose metabolism (Theodore et al., 1986a). The effect is very considerably less with phenytoin (Theodore *et al.*, 1986b). The clinical importance of this depression is uncertain, but inferences from the above-cited neuropsychological studies are tempting.

The toxic effects of clonazepam are similar to and at least as severe as those of phenobarbital. Most common are drowsiness and ataxia, as well as behavioral and personality changes (Dreifuss and Sato, 1982). Respiratory tract secretions may also increase. In a study of clonazepam in 37 patients with absence seizures, 10 could not complete the study because of side effects of the drug. Nitrazepam is less potent and may be slightly less toxic, but the reported side effects are fundamentally the same as for clonazepam (Baruzzi *et al.*, 1982). Clorazepate appears to be a typical benzodiazepine.

Somewhat less clear is the possible advantage of clobazam over the other benzodiazepines. Its molecular structure has slight but distinct structural differences from other benzodiazepines, and some epileptologists suggest that clobazam has a greater therapeutic potential and lower incidence of side effects than its close relatives (Trimble, 1986). Other experienced investigators find it to have no advantages over other benzodiazepines.

If phenobarbital must be used, its therapeutic plasma levels range from 15 to 40 µg/ml (Porter and Penry, 1980). Therapeutic primidone levels are usually in the range of 6 to 15 µg/ml. Primidone should be started at low doses and gradually increased. It is only marginally possible to obtain maximal efficacy with these drugs by increasing their plasma levels to the toxic range, as many patients have subtle toxic effects in the therapeutic range.

Anecdotal reports suggest that some antiepileptic barbiturates are preferable to others. Usually, this favoring of one barbiturate over another is based on an opinion that the favored drug has fewer side effects (especially sedation or hyperactivity) or that these side effects are somewhat less severe. All doctors who treat epileptic patients have seen occasional patients in whom the decreased toxicity of one barbiturate over another seemed convincing. Unfortunately, the hypothesis that one barbiturate is less toxic than another is especially hard to test because the majority of such drugs (except phenobarbital itself) have an active metabolite, often phenobarbital. Even if one were inclined to test clinically one drug against another, it would never be possible to eliminate the problem of a common, active metabolite with known toxic side effects. The common and uncommon barbiturates used in the United States for seizure control are shown in Table 84.1.

Phenobarbital has no known active metabolites; the principal inactive metabolite is p-hydroxyphenobarbital. Primidone (a desoxybarbiturate) is more complex. As the parent compound, it has activity comparable to that of phenobarbital, but it is also converted to phenobarbital and phenylethylmalonamide. The latter appears to have but little antiepileptic effect (Bourgeois *et al.*, 1983). The plasma phenobarbital level produced by primidone is variable; it may equal the primidone level, or more commonly (and especially in the presence of other drugs), be two or three times as high. The clinical combination of primidone and phenobarbital in a single patient has considerable potential for toxicity.

PRINCIPLE 84

Table 84.1 Antiepileptic barbiturates used in the United States

Drug	Active metabolite
Phenobarbital	None known
Primidone	Phenobarbital, phenylethylmalonamide
Mephobarbital	Phenobarbital
Metharbital	Barbital
Barbital	None known
Eterobarb (investigational)	Phenobarbital

Since primidone is rapidly converted, in large part, to phenobarbital, the effect is one of adding a metabolite when both phenobarbital and primidone are prescribed. When primidone is combined with phenytoin, enhancement of phenobarbital levels also occurs (Porro *et al.*, 1982).

Mephobarbital is converted to phenobarbital to the extent that most patients have about twenty times more phenobarbital in their plasma than they have of the parent compound (Kupferberg and Longacre-Shaw, 1979). Metharbital is changed to barbital, which in turn is apparently excreted unchanged (Maynert, 1972). Little information is available on the efficacy of this drug or its metabolite. Eterobarb, or dimethoxymethylphenobarbital, is rapidly metabolized by the liver, and although minor metabolites have been identified, the antiepileptic action of the drug can be completely explained by its conversion to phenobarbital (Goldberg, 1982).

Idiosyncratic side effects of the barbiturates include skin rashes and, much less commonly, hepatic injury. The rheumatologic effects of these drugs, probably dose related, have been underemphasized; Dupuytren's contracture and shoulder problems are surprisingly common (Mattson *et al.*, 1989).

In summary, there is little evidence that the current antiepileptic drug regimen, for most seizure types, is improved by the addition of barbiturates or benzodiazepines. There is considerable evidence that long-term use of these sedative agents has a deleterious effect. These drugs can be withdrawn, even in outpatients if done slowly and carefully. Following sedative drug withdrawal, most adults are more alert – they often say 'I didn't know how bad I felt', and most children have improved behavior.

85 Barbiturates and benzodiazepines can be withdrawn in outpatients

When the judgment has been made that a patient may profit from fewer antiepileptic drugs or when the patient is taking a barbiturate, desoxybarbiturate, or benzodiazepine, it is reasonable to consider a decrease in the sedative medications. The manner in which this adjustment can be accomplished is especially dependent on the propensity of the patient to have generalized tonic–clonic seizures; even a history of such attacks increases the risk of seizure recurrence following withdrawal (Medical Research Council Antiepileptic Drug Withdrawal Study Group, 1991). A patient with absence attacks only, and no history of generalized tonic–clonic seizures, may have drugs withdrawn with relative safety. Even if a generalized tonic–clonic seizure occurs, the likelihood of status epilepticus is minimal, especially if the patient is being treated with valproate. In a patient with frequent complex partial seizures, with secondary generalized tonic–clonic seizures every month or two, the precautions must be much more vigorous. Clearly, it is necessary to protect the patient with appropriate drugs against the occurrence of generalized tonic–clonic seizures during the withdrawal period. The most effective regimen, especially for severely affected patients, is a combination of phenytoin and carbamazepine in maximally tolerated doses, which usually means trough plasma levels of approximately 18–20 μg/ml for phenytoin and 6–7 μg/ml for carbamazepine. Status epilepticus is uncommon in patients so protected during the withdrawal period, *providing* that the withdrawal period is reasonably long. Even in patients who are seizure free for two years, two of five patients will have seizure recurrence on medication withdrawal (Medical Research Council Antiepileptic Drug Withdrawal Study Group, 1991).

The rate of withdrawal is an important aspect of antiepileptic drug discontinuation. Regardless of the long half-life of both barbiturates and benzodiazepines, a prolonged withdrawal period, with careful monitoring and frequent follow-up is the safest way of preventing serious problems. Phenobarbital withdrawal problems are greatest at the lower end of the therapeutic range; typically, few problems are encountered, for example, in dropping the plasma phenobarbital level from 60 to 30 μg/ml, but generalized tonic–clonic attacks are likely to occur as the level passes through the range of 15 to 20 μg/ml (Theodore *et al.*, 1987b). Antiepileptic drug doses should be decreased over many weeks, especially if barbiturates and benzodiazepines are being withdrawn.

It is also important to distinguish between withdrawal seizures and seizures occurring because of inadequate medication. A common error in the attempt to remove barbiturates occurs when the patient's seizures temporarily worsen and the physician assumes that the worsening indicates a need for the barbiturate rather than a withdrawal phenomenon. The result is continuation of a sedative

Table 85.1 Mean doses and plasma levels of antiepileptic drugs taken by 38 outpatients

| | Before withdrawal | | After withdrawal | |
	Dose (mg/day)	Plasma level (μg/ml)	Dose (mg/day)	Plasma level (μg/ml)
Primidone	808	7.2	0	0
Phenobarbital	115	33.2	0	0
Clonazepam	3	–	0	0
Phenytoin	309	13.5	363	18.2
Carbamazepine	1,062	4.0	1,144	6.5

From Theodore and Porter (1983b) with permission. Copyright © 1983, Wiley-Liss, Inc.

antiepileptic drug that may not be needed. In many patients it is important to try to 'weather the storm' of withdrawal; the gains may be well worth the effort.

Theodore and Porter (1983b) successfully withdrew all sedative–hypnotic drugs from 38 outpatients referred for intractable seizures. The patients ranged from 5 to 63 years of age. Withdrawal of the drugs took place over an average of twelve weeks in each patient. Primidone was the most commonly prescribed barbiturate and clonazepam the most common benzodiazepine. Withdrawal was generally well tolerated, with 11 patients reporting a transient increase in seizure frequency during the withdrawal period. Sedative–hypnotic drugs were temporarily restarted in three patients, one of whom was hospitalized for two days. Status epilepticus did not occur. At follow-up, averaging seventeen months after drug withdrawal, 32 of the patients showed improvement in either seizure frequency or medication toxicity, or both. Six patients were unchanged, but no patient was worse. Table 85.1 shows the mean doses and plasma levels of the patients' drugs before and after withdrawal of the first three. Noteworthy is the increase in the mean plasma phenytoin level from 13.5 to 18.2 μg/ml and in the mean carbamazepine level from 4.0 to 6.5 μg/ml. The largest increases in plasma levels of phenytoin and carbamazepine were accomplished early in the withdrawal period to minimize withdrawal seizures.

15 Therapy: The Role of Surgery in Epilepsy

---

86 Not everyone who has epilepsy is a surgical candidate

Surgery for epilepsy is a complex procedure which should only be performed in a center with adequate resources and experience (Consensus Panel on Surgery for Epilepsy Conference, 1990). Even if a patient has an unequivocal MRI abnormality, the relation of the epileptic focus to the anatomic lesion must be elucidated. Important resources include neuropsychological, social, and psychiatric evaluations, and patient and family education. A team approach should be used.

In the USA, there are approximately 120,000 new-onset cases of epilepsy per year (Hauser and Hesdorfer, 1990). Incidence is higher below the age of 20, and may increase in the elderly. The prevalence of active epilepsy, which includes patients who have had a seizure in the last five years or are taking AEDs, is between 6 and 7 per 1000 (Hauser and Kurland, 1975). In an British study, the lifetime prevalence of seizures was 20.2/1000, but only 5.3/1000 had 'active epilepsy' – a seizure in the last five years, or currently taking antiepileptic drugs (Goodridge and Shorvon, 1983). About 50% of the patients have partial seizures (Hauser and Kurland, 1975; Keranen *et al.*, 1988).

Some experts suggest that approximately 45% of patients with partial seizures may be 'uncontrolled' by current medications, but accurate statistics are difficult to obtain (Dreifuss, 1987). Hauser has suggested that 5–10% of patients presenting with a first unprovoked seizure each year may prove eventually to have 'non-remittent' epilepsy, but this estimate may include patients who are seizure-free or have rare seizures as long as therapeutic AED levels are maintained (Hauser and Hesdorfer, 1990).

Patients are more likely to develop intractable epilepsy if they have an abnormal neurologic exam, low IQ, psychiatric abnormalities, a history of status epilepticus, an unequivocal etiology such as head trauma, meningitis or a structural lesion (probably excluding the regions of focal gliosis now identified by increased signal intensity on MRI), secondary generalization during the first two years after seizure onset, a history of prolonged labor, febrile seizures, family history of epilepsy, CPS clusters, and/or multifocal or bilateral EEG discharges (Lindsay *et al.*, 1979; Sofijanov, 1982; Rocca *et al.*, 1987; Satischandra *et al.*, 1987; Shafer *et al.*, 1988; Smith and Dooley 1993). Seizure frequency either before or during the initial phases of AED therapy is also important. Schmidt *et al.* (1983) reported that 63% of patients with three or more complex partial and secondary generalized seizures achieved a two year remission, but seizure control occurred in only 44% of patients who had more than one generalized tonic–clonic seizure per month. Only 11% of children who had normal neurologic and neuropsychologic examinations and fewer than four seizures per year had persistent attacks on adequate AED therapy (Brorson and Wranne, 1987). However, some children experience a 'silent interval' which can last several years, during which they may be seizure-free without AEDs before intractable epilepsy develops (Lindsay *et al.*, 1984).

Unfortunately, some of the same factors associated with poor medical prognosis may also predict an unfavorable surgical outcome (Dodrill *et al.*, 1986). Patients with seizure types associated with diffuse brain dysfunction often do poorly with either surgery or AEDs. Myoclonic, atonic and 'minor motor' seizures have a particularly poor prognosis for medical therapy. Surgery may improve seizure control in patients with severe preoperative neurologic or psychiatric impairment, but fail to make a significant overall difference in a patient's life.

---

87 Reconfirm the diagnosis before surgery

The first step in identifying patients for possible surgical therapy is to confirm the diagnosis of epilepsy and to attempt to localize the onset of the seizures using video-EEG monitoring. Nonepileptic attacks, particularly psychiatric disorders, are diagnosed in 10–20% of patients admitted to monitoring units for uncontrolled epilepsy. Cardiovascular and sleep disturbances may also be misdiagnosed as epilepsy as well (Mattson, 1980). A few patients may have both pseudoseizures and epilepsy (Trimble, 1986). The physician should attempt to determine the frequency of each type of episode and the effect of each on the patient's overall function.

Once the diagnosis of epilepsy is established, the clinical seizure classification must be confirmed to make certain that the patient does not have either an unlocalized seizure disorder or one with a good prognosis. CPS are often confused with absence seizures, and other seizure types which have a good prognosis need to be identified. Perhaps the most important of these is benign rolandic epilepsy, which may be confused with partial seizures of temporal origin (Principle 16).

Experimental drug trials are an alternative to surgery. Although complete freedom from seizures is rarely accomplished with new drugs in such patients, consideration for drug trials occurs if either the patient is not enthusiastic about the prospect of surgery or the physician determines that the patient is ineligible for an operation. Since patients must be categorized according to seizure type to enter into an experimental drug trial, video-EEG monitoring is often performed before the patients are randomized. Many centers which perform surgery also enter patients into drug trials. Often, patients referred to an epilepsy center are monitored before being offered either participation in a drug trial or surgical evaluation.

---

88 Before referring a patient for surgery, make certain that the seizures are intractable

Complex partial seizure frequency in patients referred to 'intensive monitoring' units for uncontrolled epilepsy ranges from 1 per week to 5 per day (Sutula *et al.*, 1981; Theodore *et al.*, 1983b). Patients considered for corpus callosotomy may have 0–33 GTCS, but up to 500 simple partial seizures (SPS) per month (Spencer *et al.*, 1988).

Seizure frequency, although probably the most important factor, is not alone in defining intractable epilepsy. CPS vary widely in severity, duration, and in the degree of postictal confusion. Even one seizure a year will preclude obtaining a driver's license in many states/countries, and the unpredictable occurrence of even two or three seizures per year may be a significant problem for patients who are in public life or who are performing in a skilled profession.

Family members may have a significant influence on the patient's decision; in some cases the family may be more enthusiastic about surgery than the patient. Children are increasingly being referred for surgery – creating new ethical and legal issues.

Antiepileptic drugs may have adverse effects on learning and memory, especially in children – even if sedative hypnotic AEDs are not used (Hirtz and Nelson, 1985; Theodore and Porter, 1983a; Macphee *et al.*, 1986). However, the overall risks of surgery – although low – still seem greater than the risks of taking AEDs if the seizures are well-controlled. Even when patients become seizure-free, drugs are usually continued for several years post-operatively. The effect of drug withdrawal on the risk for post-operative seizure recurrence is unknown.

How many drugs should be tried before a patient is considered 'intractable'? Perhaps 40–70% of patients will obtain seizure control from either CBZ or PHT and an additional 10%–15% from these two drugs in combination (Mattson *et al.*, 1985). Valproic acid appears to be slightly less effective, but is worth a try in combination with CBZ (Mattson *et al.*, 1992). Using VPA and PHT together is more difficult because of drug interactions. A thorough trial of these three drugs would take approximately 9 months. Very few patients improve when more than two drugs are administered at a time; given the rough therapeutic equivalence of all of these drugs, the value of trying as many as three or four is questionable. Barbiturates may be useful in some patients. Although only marginally less effective, they have greater toxicity (Mattson *et al.*, 1985). Benzodiazepines are of very limited long-term value because of their neuropsychological toxicity and because of the development of tolerance.

Four new drugs are worth trying (Chapter 11). The patients entered in clinical trials of these drugs were refractory to standard agents and many could have been considered for surgery. Very few of them became seizure-free. If a patient is a good candidate, it is reasonable to try one – or at most two – of the new drugs before starting surgical evaluation.

---

89 Careful clinical and EEG studies are the basis for surgical therapy

---

All patients considered for surgery should have ictal video-EEG recordings which not only provide EEG data but which permit intensive study of the clinical seizure patterns. Certain features of the history and ictal behavior may be helpful, for example, in distinguishing temporal from frontal lobe seizure onset (Delgado-Escueta *et al.*, 1992; Williamson *et al.*, 1985; French *et al.*, 1993; Wieser and Williamson, 1993). Elementary visual sensations may reflect occipital lobe onset, whereas olfactory auras may point to the mesial temporal region. Oro-alimentary automatisms usually reflect onset in the temporal lobe, whereas short seizures with rapid secondary generalization and 'bizarre, frenetic' automatisms suggest frontal lobe origin (Wieser and Williamson, 1993).

Sphenoidal electrodes have become a routine part of the preoperative procedure in many centers (Engel *et al.*, 1990). The criteria for surface localization includes a number of factors such as the relative importance assigned to 'EEG slowing' which is contralateral to the seizure onset and the timing of appearance of contralateral discharges (Engel *et al.*, 1981; Spencer, 1981; Williamson *et al.*, 1993). About 50% of patients with CPS of temporal lobe origin can have their seizure focus localized on the basis of surface–sphenoidal EEG alone (Engel *et al.*, 1990; Theodore *et al.*, 1992; Williamson *et al.*, 1993).

There are several possible approaches to EEG localization when the surface recording is nonrevealing. Foramen ovale electrodes can detect hippocampal spikes more reliably than surface–sphenoidal recording and are associated with less risk for major complications than stereotactically placed depth electrodes

(SEEG) – although transient facial pain and dysesthesias have been reported in up to 10% of patients (Weiser *et al.*, 1993). Subdural electrodes, which can be used as either large grids or strips, are useful for functional mapping (which cannot be performed with SEEG electrodes) as well as seizure-focus localization (Luders *et al.*, 1992).

Initial studies comparing the two modalities (SEEG and subdural electrodes) in a small number of patients suggest an advantage for the former in detecting the hippocampal onset of complex partial seizures; subdural strips may not sample mesial and inferior temporal lobe as well as SEEG electrodes (Sperling and O'Connor, 1989; Spencer *et al.*, 1990). Technical issues such as number and placement of electrodes, however, may have affected the results of these studies; confirmation by more systematic investigations is needed. Since the surgery for implantation of subdural electrodes is often more extensive than for SEEG, the latter are preferable when bilateral or multifocal implantation is necessary for identification of seizure onset. A combination of both approaches can also be used in appropriate circumstances. Both kinds of electrodes have a 2–5% risk of complications such as infection or hemorrhage (the latter perhaps greater with SEEG) and increased intracranial pressure can be caused by large subdural grids (Luders *et al.*, 1992; Spencer, 1992). Spencer (1992), reviewing the literature on several hundred patients, found that 85% of patients had a good or excellent surgical outcome when the surface and depth electrode localization agreed on the locus of the abnormality, 74% did well when depth studies alone were localizing, and only 63% did well when the surface and depth localization was not in agreement.

Neuropsychological evaluation is an important part of the approach to preoperative localization, especially to establish, whenever possible, the ability of the nonresected tissue to support both language and memory after surgery. The intracarotid sodium amytal (Wada) test is often effective for speech lateralization but may be less reliable for evaluating memory function (Jones-Gotman, 1991). Transcranial magnetic stimulation may prove to be a less invasive and more easily replicable means of obtaining data on language laterality (Jennum *et al.*, 1994).

---

90 Neuroimaging tests are becoming increasingly important in the evaluation of patients for surgery

The wide availability and versatility of magnetic resonance imaging (MRI) make it ideal for evaluation of patients with epilepsy. Long TR/TE T–2 weighted sequences are preferable for revealing focal pathology – particularly mesial temporal sclerosis (MTS) and small tumors – and can correctly localize epileptic foci in up to 90% of cases (Sperling *et al.*, 1986; Theodore *et al.*, 1986c; Kuzniecky *et al.*, 1987; Jackson *et al.*, 1990). Coronal images are superior for the depiction of mesial temporal anatomy. Another approach has been to exploit the observation that hippocampal size is reduced ipsilateral to the epileptic focus, whether or not increased signal intensity is also present (Jack *et al.*, 1990; Cendes *et al.*, 1993; Ashtari *et al.*, 1991; Watson *et al.*, 1992). Measuring both the amygdala and the hippocampus (but not the anterior temporal lobe) increases the sensitivity of the procedure. Several investigators have used magnetic resonance spectroscopy to show both reduced high energy phosphate stores and the N-acetyl aspartate signal (which correlates with neuronal loss) ipsilateral to temporal lobe foci (Kuzniecky *et al.*, 1992; Hugg *et al.*, 1993).

Hippocampal atrophy also correlates with the presence of memory deficits detected by the Wada procedure and other neuropsychological tests (Lencz *et al.*, 1992; Loring *et al.*, 1993). Patients may have greater postoperative language deficits after resection of the nonatrophic left temporal lobe and greater visuospatial learning deficits after resection of the nonatrophic right temporal lobe (Trennary *et al.*, 1993). Temporal lobe tissue which is not atrophied, even though epileptogenic, may still preserve some functional reserve.

Increased signal on T2–MRI does not distinguish between small, low grade tumors, and focal gliosis (Kuzniecky *et al.*, 1987; Theodore *et al.*, 1990). Volume loss is more likely to reflect the latter, but some patients may have both an extrahippocampal foreign tissue lesion and mesial temporal sclerosis (Cascino *et al.*, 1993). Removal of both the hippocampus and the lesion may be necessary for seizure control.

Positron emission tomography with 18F-2 deoxyglucose, detects unilateral interictal temporal lobe hypometabolism (which is usually more extensive than are the structural abnormalities found on MRI) in 70–80% of patients with CPS (Engel *et al.*, 1982a; Theodore *et al.*, 1983c; Abou-Khalil *et al.*, 1987). Well-localized hypometabolism is less frequent when patients have extra-temporal EEG foci (Swartz *et al.*, 1989). Reduced metabolism is closely correlated with the presence of a histological lesion – although not always one detectable by MRI (Engel *et al.*, 1982b; Theodore *et al.*, 1990). Even in patients with mesial temporal epilepsy, hypometabolism is usually more prominent in lateral than mesial cortex (Sackellares *et al.*, 1990), perhaps because of poor spatial resolution and volume averaging, or from decreased metabolism in projection fields of dysfunctional or absent neurons. Newer scanners with improved resolution are more likely to detect hypometabolism and may be able to distinguish mesial from lateral temporal foci (Engel *et al.*, 1990; Hajek *et al.*, 1993).

'Ictal' fluorodeoxyglucose positron emission tomography (FDG-PET) scans may be performed to include interictal, ictal, and postictal metabolic phases, depending on when the seizure occurs in relation to isotope injection. In simplest terms, localized *hypo*metabolism is typically associated with interictal localization whereas localized *hyper*metabolism is typically associated with the ictal discharge. Combinations of hyper- and hypometabolic regions may be found. Both ictal and interictal PET scans should be performed with EEG and clinical monitoring to help in their interpretation (Figure 90.1).

Single photon emission computed tomography (SPECT), which measures cerebral blood flow, is easier to perform than PET because SPECT uses commercially available isotopes and does not need an on-site cyclotron. Although several tracers are available, the resolution is less than with PET.

Interictal SPECT studies show reduced interictal cerebral blood flow (CBF) in only 50% of patients with partial seizures, and false positives have been reported (Lee *et al.*, 1986; Stefan *et al.*, 1987; Rowe *et al.*, 1989). Ictal and postictal SPECT scans, feasible because of the relatively long half-life of the isotopes used, lateralize epileptic foci in 65–90%; false positives are rare. Since the results depend on the timing of isotope injection in relation to seizure onset, careful clinical and EEG monitoring is important. There is a good correlation between

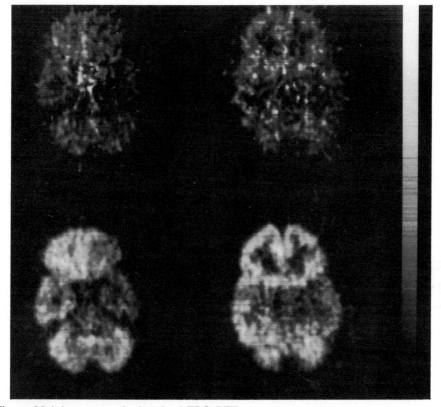

Figure 90.1 Lower panels: Interictal FDG PET scan shows pronounced right temporal hypometabolism in a patient with complex partial seizures and right mesial temporal sclerosis at surgery. Upper panels: Borderline right temporal hypoperfusion was found on an H_2 ^{15}O PET scan. Metabolism appears to be more depressed than blood flow in temporal lobe foci.

PRINCIPLE 90

ictal SPECT, MRI, and EEG localization of seizure onset (the latter using either surface ictal or depth tracings) and surgical results (Rowe *et al.*, 1989; Lee *et al.*, 1988).

Several prospective studies have shown that either hypometabolism on FDG-PET or atrophy detected by hippocampal volumetry predicts a good outcome after temporal lobectomy (Theodore *et al.*, 1992; Radke *et al.*, 1993; Cascino *et al.*, 1991; Jack *et al.*, 1992). If the hypometabolism extends outside the temporal lobe, outcome may be worse (Swartz *et al.*, 1992). When scalp–sphenoidal EEG and PET are in agreement, depth EEG studies may not provide additional information (Engel *et al.*, 1990). Since both MRI hippocampal volume loss and FDG-PET hypometabolism appear to detect the same pathophysiological process, a PET scan (or ictal SPECT) is not required if the MRI is definitely localizing. However, FDG-PET appears to be more sensitive; indeed, since some patients without increased MRI signal or hippocampal atrophy may have temporal hypometabolism on FDG-PET. Neuroimaging can also be used for functional mapping. Both PET and MRI have been used for the mapping of higher cortical function in normal volunteers (Grasby *et al.*, 1993; McCarthy *et al.*, 1993). Preliminary studies have been performed in patients with CPS of left temporal origin; these studies are in agreement with the results of subdural electrode stimulation (Bromfield *et al.*, 1991; Bookheimer *et al.*, 1993). Such techniques may become very useful for surgical planning and may replace invasive functional mapping or the Wada test in some cases.

The physician should not rely on neuroimaging techniques alone when evaluating patients for surgery (Wyllie *et al.*, 1987). A mismatch, for example, between imaging studies and surface EEG findings is an indication for invasive electrode investigations. Digital imaging techniques now allow fusion of the imaging and the invasive electrode data for surgical planning (Lemieux *et al.*, 1992) (Figure 90.2).

---

91 Temporal lobectomy is the most successful focal resection

When patients are carefully chosen for temporal lobectomy – on the basis of clinical, EEG, imaging, and neuropsychological data – the prognosis is excellent. From 60–80% can expect to be seizure-free for two years and an additional 10% have a significant reduction in seizure frequency (Engel *et al.*, 1990; Theodore *et al.*, 1992). Surgical approaches themselves vary. Some investigators advocate a 'standard' anterior temporal lobectomy. Other surgeons prefer either a tailored approach – which depends on the pre- and intraoperative evaluation and cortical

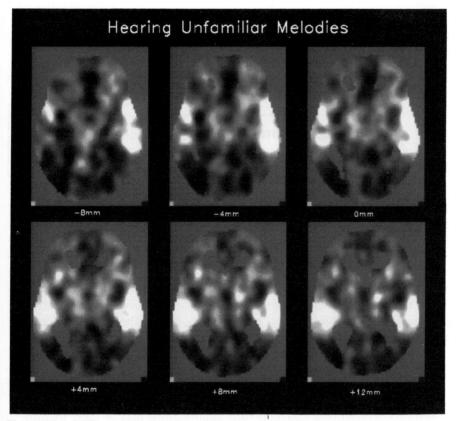

Figure 90.2 PET can be used for functional localization in patients being considered for surgery. This CBF study in a normal volunteer shows the response to hearing unfamiliar melodies. At inferior temporal levels, predominantly right-sided activation is found, while bilateral CBF increases occur at higher levels.

mapping – or a limited amygdalohippocampectomy, which may need to be followed by further surgery in some cases (Olivier, 1992). For each patient, the possibility that the more extensive surgical removal is more likely to improve outcome must be balanced against the risk of potentially greater functional loss.

Extratemporal focal resections make up 10–25% of most epilepsy surgery series (Olivier, 1990). The prognosis for postoperative seizure control is poorer than for patients with temporal lobe epilepsy, in part because of the lower reliability of localization of the ictal onset (Quesney *et al.*, 1992). Even when patients with tumors are excluded, extratemporal seizures are more likely than temporal to be associated with post-traumatic or inflammatory lesions, as well as hamartomas and cysts (Rasmussen, 1983). When unequivocal structural abnormalities are present, however, the prognosis may be improved (Olivier, 1990; Swartz *et al.*, 1989). Invasive electrode monitoring does not appear to

PRINCIPLE 91

be indicated for further localization of the seizure focus in those patients with extratemporal foci whose ictal surface EEG and imaging localization are concordant; the procedure may nevertheless be required for functional mapping (Swartz et al., 1989; Adler et al., 1991).

---

92 Hemispherectomy and corpus callosotomy may ameliorate seizures in some patients

---

Hemispherectomy is most commonly performed in children who have a severe epileptic syndrome such as Sturge–Weber, hemi-megalencephaly, or 'Rasmussen's encephalitis' (Andermann, 1992). Although most patients already have some degree of hemiparesis (which may be progressive) the potential loss of motor function must be balanced against the prospects for seizure control. Resection of the dominant hemisphere before the age of six gives the best prospects for transfer of language function (Andermann, 1992). The aim of this kind of surgery is to ameliorate seizure severity.

Patients who have frequent secondarily generalized seizures – particularly when associated with falling – but who have no unequivocal ictal focus may be considered for corpus callosotomy (Andermann, 1992). These patients often have greater neurological and neuropsychological impairment than do candidates for focal resections; also, structural abnormalities may be more frequent in this group (Purves et al., 1988). The presence of focal CT lesions or unambiguous unilateral hemispheric damage has been reported to be associated with good seizure control; if the IQ is less than 45, however, seizure control may be poor (Spencer et al., 1988; Purves et al., 1988). A postsurgical decline in language function may occur when the dominant hemisphere for speech is contralateral to the dominance for memory or handedness, perhaps because surgery disrupts the interhemispheric communication necessary for normal function in these patients (Sass et al., 1988). Unambiguous early onset CNS disease with unilateral hemispheric damage, absent memory function in the affected hemisphere and contralateral speech may predict good neuropsychologic outcome (Sass et al., 1988). When patients have no evidence of structural abnormalities, slow spike-wave discharges on EEG and ictal falls are associated with favorable clinical outcome (Gates et al., 1987; Purves et al., 1988). A more complete callosal section may be associated with better seizure control but also with greater neuropsychological impairment (Andermann, 1992).

Overall, 40–60% of these patients will have a significant reduction in seizure frequency (Reutens et al., 1993). Atonic seizures are most likely to be helped, although generalized tonic–clonic, tonic and complex partial seizures (particularly with frontal lobe origin) may be ameliorated as well (Spencer *et al.*, 1988; Reutens *et al.*, 1993).

---

93 Surgery should be considered in children as well as adults

---

One of the major goals of treatment for epilepsy is to prevent the development of the social and psychological problems experienced by many patients who have uncontrolled seizures. Success is more likely when early seizure control is obtained (Taylor, 1993). Surgery should be considered in children who have frequent seizures or whose attacks lead to disruption of school and social life; early intervention is especially relevant when the seizures do not seem to be improving and are not controlled by drugs (Blume, 1992; Shields *et al.*, 1993). Since the ultimate prognosis in children may not be as obvious as in adults, both the chance for surgical success – as defined by clinical, EEG, and imaging localization – and the risk (often low) for functional impairment, should be assessed carefully (Meyer *et al.*, 1986; Blume 1992). Children below the age of twelve may be more likely to have MRI abnormalities – particularly neuronal migration anomalies and gangliogliomas – than are older patients (Adelson *et al.*, 1992; Kuzniecky *et al.*, 1993).

Recent studies have suggested that some children with conditions such as infantile spasms or Sturge–Weber syndrome may be helped by surgery, particularly if a lesion can be identified on imaging studies (Shields *et al.*, 1993). Preliminary results are encouraging. In these children, positron emission tomography with 18F-2 deoxyglucose may be more likely to identify a dysfunctional region than is MRI (Chugani *et al.*, 1993).

The evaluation of children for surgery presents particular problems because of the difficulty of judging the impact of the disorder on the child's 'quality of life'. Parent–child interactions, both positive and negative, need to be explored; critical is the need to inquire whether the family has an agenda of its own and especially whether the family has unreasonable expectations (Taylor, 1993).

| **94** | Persistent seizures may have as much risk as surgery |

Uncontrolled epilepsy is a serious medical condition with a major impact on quality of life; it affects the ability to drive, the opportunities for obtaining employment and both social and sexual relationships. Seizure frequency may even be a factor in the intellectual decline of some patients with epilepsy. For example, patients with more frequent seizures have poorer performance on tests such as the Halstead–Reitan battery and the Wechsler Adult Intelligence Scale than do those patients whose seizures are well-controlled (Hirtz and Nelson, 1985). After surgery, improvement in employment and other measures is still related to successful seizure control (Augustine *et al.*, 1984; Dodrill, 1987).

Mortality is increased in children and adults with uncontrolled seizures (Hauser *et al.*, 1980; Lindsay *et al.*, 1979; Brorson and Wranne, 1987). Surgical mortality is less than 1% for temporal lobectomy and only 2–4% for more extensive procedures such as corpus callosotomy or hemispherectomy (Van Buren, 1987). Complications occur in about 5% of temporal lobectomies and in 11–17% of more complicated procedures. Thus, the morbidity and mortality of surgery may be no greater than that of the natural course of the uncontrolled disease.

In evaluating postsurgical deficits, mild postoperative declines in verbal memory and IQ have been reported after left temporal lobectomy whereas nonverbal deficits are seen after right temporal lobectomy (Jones-Gotman, 1987; Powell *et al.*, 1985). Function in the contralateral hemisphere, however, may improve. If seizures are controlled, the memory deficits may be ameliorated or reversed over time (Novelly *et al.*, 1984; Ojemann and Dodrill, 1985; Rausch and Crandall, 1982).

16 Therapy: Pregnancy and Epilepsy

> **95** Reevaluate all antiepileptic drugs used in pregnant epileptic patients

---

One of the most controversial subjects related to epilepsy is the proper management of pregnant epileptic patients and their offspring. In this chapter, the maternal and fetal concerns are arbitrarily separated; the maternal issues are addressed below, and the fetal issues in Principle 96.

1. Does pregnancy cause epilepsy?

Only an occasional case report confirms the occurrence of seizures limited to pregnancy (Teare, 1980). Ordinarily, pregnancy is not considered a cause of epilepsy except as a complication of other neurologic insults, such as cerebral sinus thrombosis.

2. Does pregnancy worsen epilepsy?

Available data suggest that about half the patients with epilepsy who become pregnant will have no change in their seizure frequency. Other studies show that the remaining patients are more likely to have worsening than to have improvement (Schmidt *et al.*, 1984; Bardy, 1987; Yerby, 1992). The chief factors in increased seizure frequency during pregnancy seem to be poor medication compliance and altered absorption or metabolism of drugs. Schmidt *et al.* (1984) have emphasized sleep deprivation as an important variable.

3. Does eclampsia cause epilepsy?

Although epileptic seizures may occur during severe eclampsia, there is little evidence that the seizures will persist after delivery and recovery from the metabolic disturbances.

4. Does status epilepticus occur more frequently during pregnancy?

Fortunately, there does not appear to be an increased incidence of status epilepticus during pregnancy (Schmidt, 1981; Bardy, 1987). Obviously, however, the prevention of generalized tonic–clonic status is of great importance.

5. How will pregnancy change the pharmacological action of antiepileptic drugs?

Changes may not occur at all or they may involve alterations in absorption, plasma protein binding, metabolism, and volume of distribution. If a change occurs, it is usually a fall in plasma drug levels, which return to normal after delivery. The only sure way to maintain seizure control is to monitor the plasma drug levels more frequently during pregnancy and immediately following delivery. One recent study suggests that pregnancy affects the kinetics of phenytoin much more than carbamazepine (Tomson et al., 1994).

6. Are bleeding tendencies altered by antiepileptic drug therapy?

Some evidence suggests that bleeding tendencies may be increased in neonates born to mothers taking antiepileptic drugs (Principle 96).

7. How common are compliance problems during pregnancy?

According to Schmidt (1981) and Schmidt et al. (1984) poor compliance is one of the most likely causes of increased seizures during pregnancy. Patients have problems with compliance under the best of circumstances, but with the added stress of possible teratogenic effects of the antiepileptic drugs, many patients take their drugs even less compulsively.

8. In general, what should be the physician's plan for the pregnant epileptic patient?

Overall, the physician should not change the fundamental approach to the treatment of seizures, but should monitor the patient more closely to obtain seizure control without toxicity (Yerby, 1992). For patients who are contemplating pregnancy, the physician should try to attain monotherapy and in very mild cases

Table 95.1 Recommendations for managing the pregnant epileptic patient

1. Establish a drug regimen that
   (a) gives optimal seizure control
   (b) has few side effects
   (c) requires few drugs (monotherapy is best)
   (d) does not include trimethadione or valproate

2. Make few major changes in the regimen, but
   (a) see the patient monthly
   (b) determine plasma drug levels at each visit
   (c) change the regimen only if control worsens considerably
   (d) consider the addition of vitamins with folate

3. Avoid status epilepticus by
   (a) maintaining therapeutic plasma drug levels
   (b) emphasizing patient compliance

4. Avoid toxicity after delivery by
   (a) decreasing antiepileptic drug doses slightly
   (b) following plasma drug levels closely for two to three weeks

Modified from Montouris *et al.* (1979).

even consider a trial off all medications. For the benefit of the fetus, maternal administration of folic acid, 1–5 mg/day, has been recommended (Van Allen *et al.*, 1993). Additional specific recommendations are given in Table 95.1.

---

96 Fetal abnormalities are slightly more frequent if the mother has epilepsy

The issues regarding the fetus in the pregnant epileptic patient are controversial; answers are not available to some of the most important questions. The principal issues concerning the fetus are as follows.

1. Is epilepsy inherited?

Some generalized epilepsies are hereditary. Examples are absence epilepsy, juvenile myoclonic epilepsy, and primary generalized tonic–clonic seizures. In the majority of epileptic syndromes, however, inheritance plays only a limited role; this is especially true for partial seizures. Bearing children is not to be condemned *a priori* in patients with epilepsy; the presence of sufficient genetic evidence to discourage pregnancy is very infrequent. Presumably, the father's contribution to inheritance of epilepsy is as great as the mother's. The influence of hereditary factors on fetal abnormalities is obscure and difficult to separate from the possible effects of antiepileptic drugs.

2. Do antiepileptic drugs cause fetal abnormalities?

The drugs used for epilepsy probably cause abnormalities of the fetus in a small number of pregnancies. The abnormalities are often minor, a few are severe. Of the abnormalities associated with antiepileptic drugs, the fetal hydantoin syndrome of phenytoin (Table 96.1) has been well described. However, these abnormalities may also be observed with the use of other antiepileptic drugs. The diones, trimethadione and paramethadione, are associated with a higher incidence of abnormalities than other drugs and should be avoided. Studies on valproate (Bjerkedal et al., 1982; Robert and Rosa, 1983; Lindhout et al., 1992) and on carbamazepine (Rosa, 1991) suggest an increased incidence of neural tube defects with each of these drugs, an observation which, though it requires further investigation, must be strongly considered in the choice of drugs during pregnancy. Patients who become pregnant while on either of these drugs should be counseled by their obstetrician. If one were to construct a list of antiepileptic drugs in order of their teratogenicity – and much guesswork is required – the list, from highest to lowest risk, might be: trimethadione → valproate → carbamazepine → phenytoin → phenobarbital. One recent study (Waters et al., 1994), on the other hand, rated the drugs phenobarbital → phenytoin → carbamazepine; the data on valproate were insufficient. Overall, obviously, the scientific information available is simply too poor to be certain of any conclusion.

Table 96.1 Fetal hydantoin syndrome: most common abnormalities in five children

1. Growth and performance
    (a) Motor or mental deficiency
    (b) Microcephaly
    (c) Postnatal growth deficiency

2. Craniofacial
    (a) Short nose with low nasal bridge
    (b) Hypertelorism
    (c) Low-set or abnormal ears
    (d) Short or webbed neck

3. Limb
    (a) Hypoplasia of nails and distal phalanges
    (b) Finger-like thumb

From Hanson and Smith (1975), with permission.

PRINCIPLE 96

3. Which is more likely to cause malformations – heredity or antiepileptic drugs?

No one knows the answer to this question. Although epileptic women who are not treated with antiepileptic drugs during pregnancy apparently have a lower incidence of fetal abnormalities than those who take medications (Hanson and Buehler, 1982; Kaneko *et al.*, 1992), it has been suggested that those who need medication also have increased hereditary factors. There is virtually no evidence that maternal seizures, in themselves, contribute to an increased frequency of fetal malformations.

4. Do antiepileptic drugs have a direct toxic effect on the fetus?

All antiepileptic drugs are transferred to the fetus across the placenta. Several short- and long-term effects of these drugs on the fetus have been suggested. Neonatal depression has been described, but is rarely severe and only occurs if the mother has received sedative antiepileptic drugs. Frank withdrawal symptoms in the neonate are exceedingly uncommon. The long-term effect of these drugs on brain and body development is unknown, although numerous experimental studies suggest that they may have deleterious effects. Antiepileptic drugs are transferred in breast milk to the child. Although few complications of such transfer have been described, some recommend reduced breast feeding (Kaneko *et al.*, 1981). Newborns apparently do not develop biochemical signs of osteomalacia from antiepileptic drugs (Christiansen *et al.*, 1980). Some have observed an increase in stillbirths, neonatal mortality, and neonatal jaundice in children of epileptic mothers or fathers (Janz and Beck-Mannagetta, 1981).

5. What is the overall risk of fetal abnormalities in children born to epileptic parents?

Overall, a twofold or threefold increase in the risk of fetal abnormalities is the current consensus. If the usual rate of abnormalities is considered to be 2%, then the likelihood may be 4% to 6% in such children. Parents should be counseled regarding this increased overall risk.

6. How should the newborn be managed?

Each newborn of a mother taking antiepileptic drugs should receive 1 mg of vitamin K (phytonadione) immediately after birth. Clotting factors should be monitored every two to four hours, and additional vitamin K should be administered until these factors are normal (Montouris *et al.*, 1979).

PRINCIPLE 96

17 Psychosocial Aspects of Epilepsy

97 Psychiatric disorders in people with epilepsy should be treated in the usual manner

There is an enormous literature, stretching back into the nineteenth century, on the psychiatric aspects of epilepsy (for a review, see Devinsky and Theodore, 1991). Many of the early studies, reflecting the social fears and preoccupations of their era, are more of historical than of medical interest (Temkin 1971).

Interictal personality disorders, including a wide variety of traits, have been described frequently in patients with temporal lobe foci (Devinsky, 1991). Not all studies have replicated these findings, and the medical implications are uncertain. Most of the characteristics described are accentuations of traits present in the general population. Some, such as decreased interest in sex, may be as much related to drug therapy or to chronic disease in general as to the seizures themselves (Morrell *et al.*, 1994).

Although depression may be more common in patients with epilepsy than in controls, such patients are not necessarily different from those with other chronic diseases (Altshuler, 1991). Patients with either left temporal lobe foci or inferior frontal lobe dysfunction may be more likely to be depressed (Bromfield *et al.*, 1992; Victoroff *et al.*, 1994). Patients may become more depressed, or clinically depressed for the first time, after temporal lobectomy.

The problem of evaluating psychoses in patients with epilepsy has been complicated by the failure to distinguish between ictal or postictal confusional states and interictal disorders (Schmitz and Wolf, 1991). No convincing epidemiological evidence exists to confirm clinical suspicions of an increased incidence of psychoses in patients with epilepsy. Patients who do have both epilepsy and psychosis tend to have more cerebral atrophy and focal damage than those with seizures alone (Bruton *et al.*, 1994). Some antiepileptic drugs – such as carbamazepine, ethosuximide, and particularly the new agent vigabatrin – have been reported to cause behavioral disorders, including acute psychoses, in a small number of patients.

Patients with seizures and psychiatric disease should be given the medical treatment appropriate to their psychiatric diagnosis. There is minimal evidence for seizure exacerbation caused by psychotropic medications in patients with epilepsy taking therapeutic doses of antiepileptic drugs (Ojemann *et al.*, 1987). The choice of an antidepressant or neuroleptic should depend primarily on the relative risk for sedative, anticholinergic, cardiovascular and extrapyramidal side effects.

Some psychotropic medications, such as the heterocyclic antidepressants (e.g., maprotiline), and the neuroleptics (e.g., chlorpromazine and clozapine), may be associated with an increased incidence of seizures in the general population, particularly when given at high doses (Boehnert and Lovejoy, 1985; Jabbari *et al.*, 1985; Marks and Luchins, 1991; Pies and Shader, 1994). Haloperidol and the selective serotonin reuptake blockers may be less likely to cause seizures (Marks and Luchins, 1991; Pies and Shader, 1994). The possibility of drug interactions should be kept in mind; carbamazepine, for example, induces haloperidol metabolism, and higher doses may be needed for the desired clinical effect (Fast *et al.*, 1986). Phenothiazines may reduce phenytoin and phenobarbital levels (Haidukewych and Rodin, 1985).

A most important part of the psychiatric treatment of a patient with seizures is finding a psychiatrist who understands all aspects of the disorder, and who can cooperate with the neurologist in working out a rational drug regimen – a regimen which necessarily will involve several agents with powerful central nervous system effects.

98 There may be many reasons for neuropsychological impairment in patients with epilepsy

The most important influence on cognitive function in patients with seizures is probably the underlying etiology. Patients with primary generalized epilepsy, for example, usually have normal intellectual function (Dreifuss, 1990). Even in epileptic encephalopathies associated with severe cognitive impairment, such as West's syndrome, the prognosis is better when no specific etiology can be detected.

The severity of the seizure disorder may affect cognitive function. Patients with frequent generalized tonic–clonic seizures, or with a history of status epilepticus, have a greater risk for impairment (Dodrill, 1986). In children, early seizure onset may be associated with lower cognitive function (Dam, 1990). In partial seizure disorders, the site and side of the epileptic focus may lead to specific deficits in verbal or visuospatial function and in memory (Mayeux *et al.*, 1980; Hermann *et al.*, 1987).

PRINCIPLE 98

All antiepileptic drugs probably impair cognitive function to some degree, although the effects may be difficult to measure – both because they are small and because appropriate methodology is not always used. Some investigators suggest that phenytoin has more adverse cognitive effects than other nonsedative drugs, but not everyone has confirmed this finding (Dreifuss, 1990; Aman et al., 1994). Reanalysis of a study suggesting that phenytoin was more deleterious than carbamazepine, for example, showed no difference between the drugs when blood levels were included in the analysis (Dodrill and Troupin, 1991). In another study of normal volunteers, phenytoin and carbamazepine impaired memory and performance equally (Meador et al., 1993). Barbiturates and benzodiazepines have more adverse cognitive effects than nonsedative drugs (Theodore et al., 1989b; Meador et al., 1990). Farwell et al. (1990) suggested that the adverse effect of phenobarbital might even continue after the drug had been stopped.

However, even patients who are not on antiepileptic drugs have lower performance on cognitive tests than do normal controls (Smith et al., 1986). Even stopping nonsedative drugs may lead to little improvement in some patients. Aldenkamp et al. (1993) used a broad neuropsychological test battery to study seizure-free children before and after stopping valproic acid, carbamazepine or phenytoin, and compared them to age-matched controls. Only dominant hand finger tapping showed improvement attributable to drug withdrawal.

Neurologists treating patients with epilepsy cannot (usually) modify etiology, age at onset, or seizure type. They can attempt to control seizure frequency and drug toxicity. Smaller, more frequent doses may help maintain more constant plasma levels. There is some evidence that controlled-release formulations of short half-life drugs such as carbamazepine may help to reduce adverse cognitive effects (Aldenkamp et al., 1990). Overall, patients should be given as little medication as possible and 'polytherapy' and sedative agents should be avoided. Frequent seizures, however, may be more deleterious than drugs.

---

99 People with epilepsy require a comprehensive approach to their 'quality of life'

D.C. Taylor (1979) has divided the situation of patients with chronic disease into a triad of 'disease' (for example mesial temporal sclerosis), 'illness' (recurrent seizures), and 'predicament', which encompasses the impact on the patient's life. Neurologists by the nature of their background and expertise tend to concentrate on the first two of these three aspects of epilepsy. Drugs can ameliorate the illness; surgery may cure the disease. Both therapies run the risk of leaving a patient trapped in the predicament if inadequate attention is paid to treating this last part of the triad.

Unfortunately, many people with epilepsy still consider themselves stigmatized – and indeed, many are. However, their negative self-image is related to difficulties with jobs, education, and social limitations imposed by the disorder, rather than simply by the seizures themselves. The more people learn to cope, even if seizures are not fully controlled, the better they will feel about themselves (Ryan *et al.*, 1980). Strategies for dealing with specific problems related to employment or social life may have a greater impact on the patient's quality of life than does medical treatment. Psychological counseling may be less important than job training or placement services. In some cases, specific preoperative rehabilitation planning – and even training – may do as much for the patient as the epilepsy surgery itself (Fraser *et al.*, 1993).

Driving is one of the most difficult issues faced by neurologists treating patients with seizures (Andermann *et al.*, 1988; Lipman, 1993). In defense of patients with epilepsy, factors such as age and gender may be more important than seizures in determining accident risk: women with seizures, for example, have a lower accident rate than do men who do not have epilepsy. Individual states in America vary in the seizure-free interval required to obtain a license – from 0 months (left to the physician's discretion) to 24 months. Obviously, patients with simple partial seizures that do not impair motor control, patients with only prolonged auras, or patients with predominantly nocturnal seizures may not have an increased risk for accidents. Six American states – California, Delaware, Nevada, New Jersey, Oregon, and Pennsylvania – require that physicians report their patients who have seizures to the respective department of motor vehicles.

Instruments to measure 'quality of life' have been developed for use in clinical trials of antiepileptic drugs and of surgical evaluation (Dodrill *et al.*, 1980; Jacoby *et al.*, 1992; Vickery 1993; Devinsky and Cramer, 1993). Shortened versions can be used to assess response to treatment or psychosocial intervention, as well as to highlight particular problems which need to be addressed – problems which are not apparent during routine physician–patient interactions (Devinsky, 1993).

Most important is for children and adolescents with seizures to be encouraged to perform to the limit of their abilities; any child with a chronic illness may need extra help to overcome the deleterious effects on learning of the disease and its treatment. Parents often need to be encouraged to leave the child alone; indeed, one of the greatest risks faced by a child with seizures is the parents' failure to allow the development of independence.

PRINCIPLE 99

18 The Future: The Importance of Research

> **100** We need basic research and controlled clinical trials to learn more about the treatment of epilepsy

Despite the recent introduction of four new antiepileptic drugs, it is likely that many patients will still have uncontrolled seizures or experience unacceptable adverse drug effects. We need to continue to develop new antiepileptic drugs. Drug development is a complex and expensive process which can take decades and can cost hundreds of millions of dollars. The scale of this effort creates a moral and intellectual imperative for rigorous clinical testing by clinical neurologists. Double-blind randomized clinical trials have been recognized as the standard method for proving the efficacy of new antiepileptic drugs and are required by the Food and Drug Administration – and similar organizations worldwide – before marketing. In patients with seizures, trial design is particularly important to make certain that patient and investigator bias (Porter and Malone, 1992) – as well as the intermittent and sometimes variable nature of the symptoms – do not affect the results.

To succeed, complex and expensive clinical trials need the cooperation of sponsoring organizations such as the National Institutes of Health (NIH) or industry as well as physicians and academic medical centers. Neurologists who treat patients with seizures that do not respond to current antiepileptic drugs should encourage them to consider trial participation. An interest in surgical therapy should not discourage participation in a clinical trial, as the data obtained in the pretrial evaluation may also be useful for surgical planning; the two approaches to intractable epilepsy are complementary, not exclusive.

It is ironic that surgery for epilepsy, which is becoming more popular, has not itself been evaluated by controlled trials. At this point, many neurologists believe that clinical experience validates surgery for the most common indication, uncontrolled partial seizures of temporal lobe onset, and that a formal trial would be unethical. Yet a number of aspects of surgical therapy need to be studied in formal trials. The NIH consensus conference on surgery for epilepsy identified several important questions which need answers (Consensus Panel on Surgery for Epilepsy, 1990).

The first is patient selection: at what point is a patient deemed intractable, and at what age, or after how many years of seizures, should surgery be performed? As a corollary, would patients who are seizure-free, but only on high levels of several drugs, be better off having surgery? Randomized studies could be designed to answer these questions. Although patient blinding would probably be impractical, the raters could be blinded and a statistical correction for a possible placebo effect made.

Another important area for research is the evaluation needed to identify an epileptic focus, particularly the role of depth and subdural electrodes. For procedures which have not been performed as much as temporal lobectomy – such as corpus callosotomy and hemispherectomy and even extratemporal surgery for partial seizures – the clinical benefit seems less clear and controlled trials are warranted.

Perhaps most importantly, the ideal means to assess outcome of epilepsy therapy remains uncertain. Recently, increased attention has been paid to quality of life measures – as well as to seizure frequency. The object of surgery for epilepsy is to improve the patient's life, not just reduce seizure frequency. The use of such new measures, which will be particularly valuable in comparing surgical with medical therapy, is just beginning.

We also need more information, which can only come through clinical trials, on when to start and stop treatment. Ideally, at a theoretical level, any patient with a single seizure could be entered in such a trial. There are specific problems in treating women, children, and the elderly with antiepileptic drugs that need to be studied. Some disorders occur predominantly or exclusively in children. Some drug side effects, such as phenobarbital-induced hyperactivity, may be different or more common in children.

In general, we have no cure for seizures – only more or less effective, and more or less toxic, palliative therapies. The increased interest in surgery provides an important opportunity to learn more about the neurochemistry of epilepsy. We need to know more about how and why seizures start, spread, and stop, how they affect the brain, and about the mechanisms of antiepileptic drugs. Basic research on the pathophysiology of epilepsy is essential for improvements in our ability to treat patients.

Appendix: Chapters of the International League Against Epilepsy and the International Bureau for Epilepsy

The International League Against Epilepsy (ILAE) is primarily a professional organization and the International Bureau for Epilepsy (IBE) is an organization with both lay and professional members, although it is appropriately dominated by the former. The purpose of this appendix is to guide physicians to expertise in epilepsy in their various countries through the ILAE and IBE chapters. This list, provided by each organization, is accurate as of mid-1994. Publication of the list does not in any way imply endorsement of this volume by ILAE or IBE or their various chapters.

ALGERIA

(ILAE)
President, Algerian League Against
   Epilepsy
Service de Neurologie
C H U Mustapha
16000 Alger

ARGENTINA

(IBE)
Ass. de Lucha Contra la Epilepsia
Tucuman 3261
1425 Buenos Aires

(ILAE)
Presidente L.A.C.E.
a/c Sociedad Neurologica Argentina
Combate de los Pozos 59
Piso 1, Depto. 5
1079 Buenos Aires

AUSTRIA

(IBE)
Elterninitiative fur Anfallskranke Kinder
Stumpergasse 1/15
1060 Wien

(ILAE)
1. Vorsitzender
Osterrreichische Sektion der
   Internationalen Liga Gegen Epilepsie
Neurologische Universitatsklinik
Auenbruggerplatz 22
A-8036 Graz

AUSTRALIA

(IBE)
Nat. Epilepsy Assn. of Australia
PO Box 224,
Parramatta NSW 2150

(ILAE)
President, Epilepsy Society of Australia
Department of Neurology
Austin Hospital
Heidelberg, Vic. 3084

BELGIUM

(IBE)
Belg. Nat. Bond Tegen Epilepsie
Avenue Albert 135
Brussels 1060

BRAZIL

(ILAE)
Presidente, Liga Brasileira de Epilepsia
(LBE)
UNICAMP-Cx. Postal: 6138
CEP: 13081-970
Campinas-SP

BULGARIA

(ILAE)
Bulgarian Association Against Epilepsy
Institute for Pediatrics
11D Nestorov
Sofia 1606

BURKINA FASO

(ILAE)
President, Ligue Burkinabe Contre
l'Epilepsie (LBCE)
01 BP 2317
Ouagadougou 01
Province du Kadiogo
Burkina Faso

CANADA

(IBE)
Epilepsy Canada
1470 Peel Street, suite 745
Montreal, Quebec H3A 1T1

(ILAE)
President, Canadian League Against
Epilepsy
Victoria General Hospital
1278 Tower Road, Room 2150 ACC
Halifax, Nova Scotia B3H 2Y9

CHILE

(IBE)
Ass. Liga contra la Epilepsia de
Valparaiso
PO Box 705
Vina del Mar

(ILAE)
Presidente, Liga Chilena contra la
Epilepsia
Patriotas Uruguayos 2236 (ex Los
Ceibos)
Santiago

COLOMBIA

(IBE)
Liga Colombiana contra la Epilepsia
PO Box 057751
Bogota DC

(ILAE)
Director, Fundacion Liga Gentral Contra
la Epilepsia
Calle 35, N 17–48
Bogota, D.E.
Colombia

CUBA

(IBE)
Ministerio se Salud Publica
Inst. Neurol/Neurochir. 29 yD, aptdo.
4248 Vedado
Havana 4 10400

(ILAE)
Presidente, Liga Cubana contra la
Epilepsia
Instituto de Neurologia y Neurocirugia
Zona Postal 4, Apartado 4248
C. Habana 10400

CZECH REPUBLIC

(ILAE)
Clinic of Pediatric Neurology
2nd Medical Faculty
Charles University
V uvalu 84
15018 Prague 5-Motol

DENMARK

(IBE)
Dansk Epilepsiforening,
Dr. Sellsvej 28
DK 4293 Dianalund

(ILAE)
University Clinic of Neurology
Hvidovre Hospital
DK-2650 Hvidovre

DOMINICAN REPUBLIC

(ILAE)
Tte. Amado Garcia Querrero No. 233
Santo Domingo

ECUADOR

(IBE)
Asoc. de Padres de Ninos con Epilepsia
PO Box 17-15-221 C
Quito

(ILAE)
Liga Ecuatoriana Contra la Epilepsia
Clinica Internacional
Av. America 3520
Quito

FINLAND

(IBE)
Epilepsyaliitto
Kalevankatu 61
00180 Helsinki 18

(ILAE)
President, Finnish Epilepsy Society
Department of Child Neurology
University of Turku
University Hospital TYKS
SF-20520 Turku

FRANCE

(IBE)
A.I.S.P.A.C.E.
11 Avenue Kennedy
F-59800 Lille

(ILAE)
President, Ligue Francaise contre
    l'Epilepsie
Centre Hospitalier Lyon-Sud 3B
F-69310 Pierre-Benite

GERMANY

(IBE)
Deutsche Epilepsie Vereinigung
Sulzaer Str. 5
14199 Berlin

(ILAE)
1. Vorsitzender
Deutsche Sektion der Internationalen Liga
    gegen Epilepsie
Institut f. Physiologie der Charite
Abteilung Neurophysiologie
Hessische Str. 3–4
D-10115 Berlin

GREAT BRITAIN (see also Scotland)

(IBE)
British Epilepsy Association
Antsey House, 40 Hanover Square
Leeds L53 1BE

(ILAE)
Nat. Hospital for Nervous Diseases
Queen Square
London WC1N 3BG

GREECE

(IBE)
Greek Nat. Assn. Against Epilepsy, Aghia
  Sophia
Children's Hospital, Dept. of
  Neur./Neurophys.
Athens 11527

GUATEMALA

(IBE)
Guatemalan Epilepsy Society,
  CAGUALICE
Av. La Reforma 1–64, Zona 9

(ILAE)
CAGUALICE, Liga Internacional contra
  la Epilepsia
Capitulo Guatemala
Av. La Reforma 1–64, zona 9

HUNGARY

(ILAE)
Hungarian Chapter of the International
  League against Epilepsy
PO Box 1
H-1261 Budapest 27

INDIA

(IBE)
Indian Epilepsy Association
nr. 1 Old Veterinary Hospital Road
Basavanagudi Bangalore 560 004

(ILAE)
Indian Epilepsy Association
1, Old, Veterinary Hospital Road
Basavanagudi
Bangalore 560 004

INDONESIA

(IBE)
PERPEI,
Jl. Jelita Utara no. 11, Rawamangun
Jakarta 13220

(ILAE)
The Indonesian Society Against Epilepsy
c/o Bag. Neurologi F.K.U.I./R.S.C.M.
Jl. Salemba 6
Jakarta

IRELAND

(IBE)
Irish Epilepsy Association
249 Crumlin Road
Dublin 12

ISRAEL

(IBE)
Israel Epilepsy Association
4 Avodat Yisrael St., PO Box 1598
Jerusalem

(ILAE)
President, Israeli Chapter of the
   International League Against Epilepsy
Dept. of Neurology
Western Galilee Regional Hospital -
   Nahariya
PO Box 21
Nahariya 22100

ITALY

(IBE)
Italian chapter of IBE, c/o Studio
   Lamattina-Frumento
Via Assarotti 44/4
16 122 Genoa

(ILAE)
Presidente, Lega Italiana contro l'Epliessia
Cattedra di Neuropsichiatria Infantile
Ploiclinico Borgo Roma
1–37134 Verona

JAPAN

(IBE)
The Japanese Epilepsy Association
5F Zenkokuzaiden Building 2-2-8,
   Nishiwaseda
Shinjuku-Ku
Tokyo 162

(ILAE)
President, Japan Epilepsy Society
c/o National Epilepsy Center
Shizuoka Higashi Hospital
886 Urushiyama, Shizuoka 420

KENYA

(IBE)
Kenya Ass. f/t Welfare of Epileptics,
Gertrude's Garden, Childrens Hospital,
   PO Box 42325
Nairobi

KOREA

(IBE)
Korean Epilepsy Association
204-1 Yeonhi-dong, Seodaemun-ku
Seoul 120-112

MEXICO

(IBE)
'Group "Acceptation" of Epileptics'
Amsterdam 1928 #19, Colonia Olimpica-
   Pedregal
Mexico 04710 D.F.

(ILAE)
Capitulo Mexicano de la Liga
   Internacional Contra la Epilepsia
Eclipse 2745
J. del Bosque
C.P. 44520
Guadalajara, Jal.

MOROCCO

(ILAE)
Ligue marocaine contre l'Epilepsie
Hopital des Specialites
Rabat

THE NETHERLANDS

(IBE)
Epilepsie Vereniging Nederland,
PO Box 9587
3506 GN Utrecht

(ILAE)
Chairman, Nederlandse Liga tegen
   Epilepsie
Pahud de Martangesdreef 61
NL–3562 AB Utrecht

NEW ZEALAND

(IBE)
Epilepsy Association of New Zealand Inc.
PO Box 1074
Hamilton

NORWAY

(IBE)
Norsk Epilepsiforbund,
Storgt. 39
0192 Oslo

(ILAE)
President, Norwegian Chapter of the
    International League against Epilepsy
Statens Senter for Epilepsi
PO Box 900
N-1301 Sandvika

PANAMA

(ILAE)
Presidente, Liga Panamena Contra la
    Epilepsia
Apartado Postal 6-8250
El Dorado, Panama
Republica de Panama

PERU

(ILAE)
Secretaria General de la Liga Peruana
    Contra la Epilepsia
Avenida 2 de Mayo 649
San Isidro-Lima
Peru

POLAND

(IBE)
Polish Epilepsy Association
15–482 Bialystok
Ul. Fabryczna 57 (XIp.pok.7)

(ILAE)
President, Polish League Against Epilepsy
Dept. of Neurology and Epileptology
Medical Center for Postgraduate
    Education
ul. Czerniakowska 231
00-416 Warsawa

PORTUGAL

(IBE)
Liga Nac. Portug. c.l. Epilepsia
Rua Sa da Bandeira 162–1 o
4000 Porto

(ILAE)
President, Liga Portuguesa Contra a
    Epilepsia
R. Sa da Bandeira 162, 1
4000 Porto

RUSSIA

(ILAE)
President of the Russian League Against
    Epilepsy
Academy of Medical Sciences
Solaynka str. No. 14
117049 Moscow
Russia

SCOTLAND

(IBE)
Epilepsy Assn. of Scotland
48 Govan Road
Glasgow G51 1J1

SLOVENIA

(IBE)
Liga Proti Epilepsiji
CIPD, Njegoseva 4/11
61 000 Ljubljana

(ILAE)
Slovenian League Against Epilepsy
Njegoseva 4
61104 Ljubljana
Slovenia

SOUTH AFRICA

(IBE)
South Africa Nat. Epilepsy League,
　S.A.N.E.L.
PO Box 73
Observatory 7935

SPAIN

(IBE)
P.E.N.E.P.A.
Calle Escuelas Pias n. 89
Barcelona 08017

(ILAE)
Presidente, Liga Espanola Contra la
　Epilepsia
Neuropediatria
Hospital Univ. Valdecilla
39008 Santander

SRI LANKA

(IBE)
Epilepsy Assn. of Sri Lanka
10 Austin Place
Colombo 8

SWEDEN

(IBE)
Swedish Epilepsy Association
PO Box 9514
10274 Stockholm

(ILAE)
President, Swedish Epilepsy Society
Neur. klin.
Karolinska Sjukhuset
Box 60 500
S-104 01 Stockholm

SWITZERLAND

(IBE)
Schweiz Liga gegen Epilepsie
c/o Pro Infirmis, Postfach 129
8032 Zurich

(ILAE)
Prasident, Schweizerische Liga gegen
　Epilepsie (SLgE)
Universitatsspital Zurich
Neurologische Klinik
Frauenklinikstr. 26
CH-8006 Zurich

TAIWAN

(ILAE)
President, Chinese Epilepsy Society
c/o Dept. of Neurology
National Cheng Kung University
Medical Center
138-Sheng-Li Road
Tainan 704

TURKEY

(ILAE)
President, Epilepsy Society of Turkey
c/o 1-7-C-27 7-8. Kisim Atakoy
34750 Istanbul
Turkey

USA

(IBE)
Epilepsy Foundation of America
4351 Garden City Drive
Landover, Maryland 20785

(ILAE)
President, American Epilepsy Society
638 Prospect Avenue
Hartford, Connecticut 06105

URUGUAY

(ILAE)
Liga Uruguaya contra la Epilepsia
Hospitalde Clinicas, Piso 2
Av. Italia s/n
11600 Montevideo

VENEZUELA

(ILAE)
Presidente, Liga Venezolana Contra La
  Epilepsia
Quebrada Honda a Santa Rosa
Edificio Tachira, Planta Baja
C.P. 1050 Caracas

YUGOSLAVIA

(ILAE)
President of the Yugoslav Union of
  Leagues against Epilepsy
Institute of Mental Health
Palmoticeva 37
1100 Beograd

ZAIRE

(ILAE)
Ligue Zairoise Contre l'Epilepsie
c/o Centre Neuropsycho-pathologique
B/P/ 825
Kinshasa XI

ZIMBABWE

(IBE)
Epilepsy Support Foundation
PO Box A. 104
Avondale, Harare

Bibliography

Abou-Khalil BW, Siegel GJ, Sackellares JC et al. (1987) Positron emission tomography studies of cerebral glucose metabolism in chronic partial epilepsy. *Ann Neurol* **22**, 480–486.

Abou-Khalil B, Andermann E, Andermann F, Olivier A and Quesney LF (1993) Temporal lobe epilepsy after prolonged febrile convulsions: excellent outcome after surgical treatment. *Epilepsia* **34**, 878–887.

Adams RD and Foley JM (1953) The neurological disorder associated with liver disease. *Proceedings of the Association for Research in Nervous and Mental Disease*, **32**, 198–237.

Adelson PD, Peacock WJ, Chugani HT, Comair YG, Vinters HG, Shields WD and Shewmon DA (1992) Temporal and extended temporal resections for the treatment of intractable seizures in early childhood. *Pediatr Neurosurg* **18**, 169–178.

Adler J, Erba G, Winston KR et al. (1991) Results of surgery for extratemporal partial epilepsy that began in childhood. *Arch Neurol* **48**, 133–140.

Aicardi J and Chevrie JJ (1983) Consequences of status epilepticus in infants and children. In Delgado-Escueta AV, Wasterlain CG, Treiman DM and Porter RJ (Eds) *Advances in Neurology, Vol 34: Status Epilepticus – Mechanisms of Brain Damage and Treatment*. New York: Raven Press, pp. 115–125.

Albani F, Riva R, Contin M and Baruzzi A (1992) A within subject analysis of carbamazepine disposition related to development in children with epilepsy. *Ther Drug Monit* **14**, 457–460.

Aldenkamp AP, Alpherts MC, Moerland N, Ottevanger N and Van Parys JAP (1987) Controlled release carbamazepine. Cognitive side effects in patients with epilepsy. *Epilepsia* **28**, 507–514.

Aldenkamp AP, Alpherts WCJ, Dekker MCA and Overweg J (1990) Neuropsychological aspects of learning disabilities in epilepsy. *Epilepsia* **31** (Suppl 4), 9–20.

Aldenkamp AP, Alpherts WCJ, Blennow G, Elmqvist D, Heijbel J, Nilsson HL, Sandstedt P, Tonnby, B, Wahlander L and Wosse E (1993) Withdrawal of antiepileptic medication in children – effects on cognitive function: the multicenter Holmfrid study. *Neurology* **43**, 41–50.

Alldredge BK and Lowenstein DH (1993) Status epilepticus related to alcohol abuse. *Epilepsia* **34**, 1033–1037.

Altshuler L (1991) Depression and epilepsy. In Devinsky O and Theodore WH (Eds) *Epilepsy and Behavior*. New York: Wiley-Liss, pp. 47–66.

Aman MG, Werry JS, Paxton JW and Turbott SH (1994) Effects of phenytoin on cognitive-motor performance in children as a function of drug concentration, seizure type, and time of medication. *Epilepsia* **35**, 172–180.

American Psychiatric Association (1993) DSM-IV Draft Criteria (for the *Diagnostic and Statistical Manual of Mental Disorders*). Washington, DC: American Psychiatric Press, pp. N1–N3.

REFERENCES

Aminoff MJ and Simon RP (1980) Status Epilepticus: causes, consequences, and clinical features in 98 patients. *Am J Med* **69**, 657–666.

Aminoff MJ, Scheinman MM, Griffin JC and Herre JM (1988) Electrocerebral accompaniments of syncope associated with malignant ventricular arrhythmias. *Annals of Internal Medicine* **108**, 791–796.

Andermann F and Robb JP (1972) Absence status: A reappraisal following review of thirty-eight patients. *Epilepsia* **13**, 177–187.

Andermann F, Remillard GM, Zifkin BG, Trottier AG and Drouin P (1988) Epilepsy and driving. *Can J Neurol Sci* **15**, 371–377.

Andermann F (1992) Clinical indications for hemispherectomy and callosotomy. In Theodore WH (Ed.) *Surgical Treatment of Epilepsy. Epilepsy Research Suppl 5*. Amsterdam: Elsevier, pp. 189–199.

Andermann F (1993) Non-epileptic paroxysmal neurologic events. In Rowan JA and Gates JR (Eds) *Non-Epileptic Seizures*. Boston: Butterworth-Heinemann, pp. 111–121.

Annegers JF, Grabow JD, Groover RV, Laws ER, Elveback LR and Kurland LT (1980) Seizures after head trauma: A population study. *Neurology* **30**, 683–689.

Annegers JF, Shirts SB, Hauser WA and Kurland LT (1985) Risk of recurrence after an initial unprovoked seizure. *Epilepsia* **27**, 43–50.

Annegers JF, Hauser WA, Shirts SB and Kurland LT (1987) Factors prognostic of unprovoked seizures after febrile convulsions. *N England J of Med,* **316**, 493–498.

Artieda J and Obeso JA (1993) The pathophysiology and pharmacology of photic cortical reflex myoclonus. *Ann Neurol* **34**, 175–184.

Arts WFM, Visser LH, Loonen MCB, Tjiam AT, Stroink H, Stuurman PM and Poortvliet DCJ (1988) Follow-up of 146 children with epilepsy after withdrawal of antiepileptic therapy. *Epilepsia* **29**, 244–250.

Asconape J and Penry JK (1984) Some clinical and EEG aspects of benign juvenile myoclonic epilepsy. *Epilepsia* **25**, 108–114.

Asconape JJ, Penry JK, Dreifuss FE, Riela A and Mirza W (1993) Valproate-associated pancreatitis. *Epilepsia* **34**, 177–183.

Asconape JJ, Manning KR and Lancman ME (1994) Systemic lupus erythematosus associated with use of valproate. *Epilepsia* **35**, 162–163.

Ashtari M, Barr WB, Schaul N and Bogerts B (1991) Three-dimensional fast low-angle shot imaging and computerized volume measurement of the hippocampus in patients with chronic epilepsy of the temporal lobe. *AJNR* **12**, 941–994.

Augustine E, Novelly RA, Mattson RH *et al.* (1984) Occupational adjustment following neurosurgical treatment of epilepsy. *Ann Neurol* **15**, 68–72.

Bagby GC (1988) Leukopenia. In Wyngaarden JB and Smith LH (Eds) *Textbook of Medicine*. Philadephia: WB Saunders, pp. 961–967.

Bardy AH (1987) Incidence of seizures during pregnancy, labor and puerperium in epileptic women: A prospective study. *Acta Neurol Scand* **75**, 356–360.

Barre J, Didey F, Delion F and Tillment JP (1988) Problems in therapeutic drug monitoring: free level drug monitoring. *Ther Drug Monit* **10**, 133–143.

Barry E and Hauser WA (1993) Status epilepticus: the interaction of epilepsy and acute brain disease. *Neurology* **43**, 1473–1478.

Barry E and Hauser WA (1994) Status epilepticus and antiepileptic medication levels. *Neurology* **44**, 47–50.

Baruzzi A, Michelucci R and Tassinari CA (1982) Benzodiazepines: Nitrazepam. In Woodbury DM, Penry JK and Pippenger CE (Eds) *Antiepileptic Drugs* (second edition). New York: Raven Press, pp. 753–769.

Beaussart M and Faou R (1978) Evolution of epilepsy with rolandic paroxysmal foci: A study of 324 cases. *Epilepsia* **19**, 337–342.

Bender AD (1968) Effect of age on intestinal absorption: implications for drug absorption in the elderly. *J Am Geriatr Soc* **16**, 1331–1339.

Ben Menachem E, Persson LI, Schechter PJ, Haegele KD and Huebert N (1988) Effects of single doses of vigabatrin on CSF concentrations of GABA, homocarnosine, homo-vanillic acid, and 5-hydroxyindoleacetic acid in patients with complex partial epilepsy. *Epilepsy Research* **2**, 96–101.

Berg AT and Shinnar S (1991) The risk of seizure recurrence after a first unprovoked seizure: a quantitative review. *Neurology* **41**, 965–972.

Berg AT and Shinnar S (1994) Relapse following discontinuation of antiepileptic drugs: a meta-analysis. *Neurology* **44**, 601–608.

Berg AT, Shinnar S, Hauser WA *et al.* (1992) A prospective study of recurrent febrile seizures. *N Engl J Med* **327**, 1122–1127.

Berkovic S, Andermann F, Carpenter S and Wolfe LS (1986) Progressive myoclonus epi-lepsies: specific causes and diagnosis. *N Engl J Med* **315**, 296–305.

Bertilsson L, Hojer B, Tybring G, Osterloh J and Rane A (1980) Autoinduction of carba-mazepine metabolism in children examined by a stable isotope technique. *Clin Pharm-acol Ther* **27**, 83–88.

Bialer M (1992) Pharmacokinetic evaluation of sustained release formulations of antiepi-leptic drugs. Clinical Implications. *Clin Pharmacokinet* **22**, 11–21.

Bialer M (1993) Comparative pharmacokinetics of the newer antiepileptic drugs. *Clin Pharmacokinet* **24**, 441–452.

Binnie CD (1989) Potential antiepileptic drugs: flunarizine and other calcium entry block-ers. In Levy RH, Dreifuss FE, Mattson RH, Meldrum BS and Penry JK (Eds) *Antiepi-leptic Drugs*. New York: Raven Press, pp. 971–182.

Binnie CD, Debets RMC, Engelsman M, Meijer JWA, Meinardi H, Overweg J, Peck AW, Van Wieringen A and Yuen WC (1989) Double-blind crossover trial of lamotrigine (Lamictal) as add-on therapy in intractable epilepsy. *Epilepsy Res* **4**, 222–229.

Bjerkedal T, Czeizel A, Goujard J, Kallen B, Mastroiacova P, Nevin N, Oakley G and Robert E (1982) Valproic acid and spina bifida. *Lancet* **2**, 1096.

Blomquist HK and Zetterlund B (1985) Evaluation of treatment in typical absence seiz-ures. The role of long-term EEG monitoring and ethosuximide. *Acta Paediatr Scand* **74**, 409–415.

Blume WT (1987) Lennox–Gastaut Syndrome. In Luders H and Lesser R (Eds) *Epilepsy: Electroclinical Syndromes*. Heidelberg: Springer-Verlag, pp. 73–92.

Blume WT (1992) Uncontrolled Epilepsy in children. In Theodore WH (Ed.) *Surgical Treatment of Epilepsy. Epilepsy Research Suppl 5*. Amsterdam: Elsevier, pp. 19–24.

Boehnert MT and Lovejoy FH (1985) Value of the QRS duration versus the serum drug level in predicting seizures and ventricular arrhythmias after an acute overdose of tri-cyclic antidepressants. *N Engl J Med* **313**, 474–479.

Bonneton J, Iliadis A, Genton P, Dravet C, Viallet D and Mesdjian E (1993) Steady-state pharmacokinetics of conventional versus controlled-release carbamazepine in patients with epilepsy. *Epilepsy Res* **14**, 257–263.

Booker HE and Darcey B (1973) Serum concentrations of free diphenylhydantoin and their relationship to clinical intoxication. *Epilepsia* **14**, 177–184.

Bookheimer SY, Zeffiro TA, Theodore W, Malow B, Blaxton T, Sato S and Gaillard W (1993) Multimodality functional imaging for language localization in Epilepsy. *Neur-ology* **43** (Suppl), A193.

REFERENCES

Bourgeois BFD, Dodson WE and Ferrendelli JA (1983) Primidone, phenobarbital, and PEMA: Seizure protection, neurotoxicity, and therapeutic index of individual compounds in mice. *Neurology* 33, 283–290.

Bourgeois B, Leppik IE, Sackellares JC *et al.* (1993) Felbamate: a double-blind controlled trial in patients undergoing presurgical evaluation of partial seizures. *Neurology* 43, 693–696.

Bouma PAD, Peters ACB, Arts RJHM, Stijnen Th and Van Rossum J (1987) Discontinuation of antiepileptic therapy: a prospective study in children. *J Neurol Neurosurg Psychiatr* 50, 1579–1583.

Bowden CL, Brugger AM, Swann AC, Calabrese JR, Janicak PG, Petty F, Dilsaver SC, Davis JM, Rush AJ, Small JG, Garza-Trevino ES, Risch SC, Goodnick PJ and Morris DD (1994) Efficacy of divalproex vs lithium and placebo in the treatment of mania. *J Am Med Assoc* 271, 918–924.

Bowdle TA, Patel IH, Levy RH and Wilensky AJ (1980) Valproic acid dosage and plasma protein binding and clearance. *Clin Pharmacol Ther* 28, 486–492.

Brent DA, Crumrine PK, Varma RR, Allan M and Allman C (1987) Phenobarbital treatment and major depressive disorder in children with epilepsy. *Pediatrics* 80, 909–917.

Brodie MJ, Forrest G and Rapeport WG (1983) Carbamazepine 10, 11 epoxide concentrations in epileptics on carbamazepine alone and in combination with other anticonvulsants. *Br J Clin Pharmacol* 16, 747–750.

Bromfield EB, D'Ambroisa J, Devinsky O, Nice FJ and Theodore WH (1989) Phenytoin withdrawal and seizure frequency. *Neurology* 39, 905–909.

Bromfield EB, Ludlow CL, Sedory S, Leiderman DB and Theodore WH (1991) Cerebral activation during speech perception in temporal lobe epilepsy. *Epilepsy Research* 9, 49–58.

Bromfield EB, Altshuler LL, Leiderman DB, Balish MN, Ketter TA, Devinsky O, Post RM and Theodore WH (1992) Cerebral metabolism and depression in patients with complex partial seizures. *Arch Neurol* 49, 617–625.

Brorson LO and Wranne L (1987) Long-term prognosis in childhood epilepsy: survival and seizure prognosis. *Epilepsia* 28, 324–330.

Brown P, Day BL, Rothwell JC, Thompson PD and Marsden CD (1991) Intrahemispheric and interhemispheric spread of cerebral cortical myoclonic activity and its relevence to epilepsy. *Brain* 114, 2333–2351.

Browne TR, Penry JK, Porter RJ and Dreifuss FE (1974) Responsiveness before, during, and after spike-wave paroxysms. *Neurology* 24, 659–665.

Browne TR, Dreifuss FE, Dyken PR, Goode DJ, Penry JK, Porter RJ, White BG and White PT (1975) Ethosuximide in the treatment of absence (petit mal) seizures. *Neurology* 25, 515–524.

Browne TR, Feldman RG and Buchanan RA (1983) Methsuximide for complex partial seizures: efficacy, toxicity, clinical pharmacology, and drug interactions. *Neurology* 33, 414–418.

Browne TR, Mattson RH, Penry JK *et al.* (1987) Vigabatrin for complex partial seizures: multicenter single-blind study with long-term follow-up. *Neurology* 37, 184–189.

Browne TR, Szabo GK, Evans JE, Evans BA, Greenblatt DJ and Mikati MA (1988) Carbamazepine increases phenytoin serum concentration and reduces phenytoin clearance. *Neurology* 38, 1146–1150.

Browne TR and Chang Tsun (1989) Phenytoin: biotransformation. In Levy R, Mattson R, Meldrum B, Penry JK and Dreifuss FE (Eds) *Antiepileptic Drugs* (third edition). New York: Raven Press, pp. 197–213.

Bruni J and Albright P (1983) Valproic acid as therapy for complex partial seizures: its efficacy and toxic effects. *Arch Neurol* **40**, 135–137.

Bruton CJ, Stevens JR and Frith CD (1994) Epilepsy, psychosis, and schizophrenia: clinical and neuropathologic correlations. *Neurology* **44**, 34–42.

Buchthal F and Svensmark O (1959–60) Aspects of the pharmacology of phenytoin (Dilantin) and phenobarbital relevent to their dosage in the treatment of epilepsy. *Epilepsia* **1**, 373–384.

Buchthal F, Svensmark O and Schiller PJ (1960) Clinical and electroencephalographic correlation with serum levels of diphenylhydantoin. *Arch Neurol* **2**, 624–630.

Callaghan N, Kenny RA, O'Neill B, Crowley M and Goggin T (1985) A prospective study between carbamazepine, phenytoin, and sodium valproate as monotherapy in previously untreated and recently diagnosed patients with epilepsy. *J Neurol Neurosurg Psychiatr* **48**, 639–644.

Callaghan N, Garrett A and Goggin T (1988) Withdrawal of anticonvulsant drugs in patients free of seizures for two years. *N Engl J Med* **318**, 942–946.

Camfield PR, Camfield CS, Dooley JM, Smith E and Garner B (1989) A randomized study of carbamazepine versus no medication after a first unprovoked seizure in childhood. *Neurology* **39**, 851–852.

Cascino GD, Hirschorn KA, Jack CR and Sharbrough FW (1989) Gadolinium-DTPA-enhanced magnetic resonance imaging in intractable partial epilepsy. *Neurology* **39**, 1115–1118.

Cascino GD, Jack CR, Parisi J *et al.* (1991) Magnetic resonance image-based volume studies in temporal lobe epilepsy: pathological correlations. *Ann Neurol* **30**, 31–36.

Cascino GD (1993) Nonconvulsive status epilepticus in adults and children. *Epilepsia* **34** (Suppl 1), S21–S28.

Cascino GD, Jack CR, Parisi JE, Sharbrough FW, Schreiber CP, Kelly PJ and Trennerry MR (1993) Operative strategy in patients with MRI-identified dual pathology and temporal lobe epilepsy. *Epilepsy Res* **14**, 175–182.

Cendes F, Andermann F, Gloor P *et al.* (1993) MRI volumetric measurement of amygdala and hippocampus in temporal lobe epilepsy. *Neurology* **43**, 719–725.

Chadwick DW (1985) Concentration-effect relationships of valproic acid. *Clin Pharmacokin* **10**, 155–163.

Chadwick DW (1987) Valproate monotherapy in the management of generalized and partial seizures. *Epilepsia* **28** (Suppl 2), S12–S17.

Chang T (1989) Ethosuximide: absorption, distribution, and excretion. In Levy R, Mattson R, Meldrum B, Penry JK and Dreifuss FE (Eds) *Antiepileptic Drugs* (third edition). New York: Raven Press.

Charleton MH (Ed.) (1975) *Myoclonic Seizures*. Amsterdam: Exerpta Medica. 167 pp.

Chauvel P, Louvel J and Lamarche M. (1978) Transcortical reflexes and focal motor epilepsy. *EEG Clin Neurophysiol* **45**, 309–318.

Christiansen C, Brandt NJ, Ebbesen F, Sardemann H and Trolle D (1980) Do newborns of epileptics on anticonvulsants develop biochemical signs of osteomalacia? A controlled prospective study. *Acta Neurol Scand* **62**, 158–164.

Chugani HT, Mazziotta JC, Engel J and Phelps ME (1987) The Lennox–Gastaut syndrome: Metabolic subtypes determined by 2-deoxy-2–18F-fluoro-D-glucose positron emission tomography. *Ann Neurol* **21**, 4–13.

Chugani HT, Shewmon DA, Shields WD *et al.* (1993) Surgery for intractable infantile spasms: neuroimaging perspectives. *Epilepsia* **34**(4), 764–771.

REFERENCES

Clancy RR, Legido AL and Lewis D (1988) Occult neonatal seizures. *Epilepsia* **29**, 256–261.

Cloyd JC and Kriel RL (1981) Bioavailability of rectally administered valproic acid syrup. *Neurology* **31**, 1348–1352.

Cloyd JC, Kriel RL, Fischer JH, Sawchuk RJ and Eggerth RM (1983) Pharmacokinetics of valproic acid in children: 1. Multiple antiepileptic drug therapy. *Neurology* **33**, 185–191.

Cloyd J (1991) Pharmacokinetic pitfalls of present antiepileptic medications. *Epilepsia* **32** (Suppl 5), 53–65.

Cochran EB, Massey KL, Phelps SJ, Cramer JA, Toftness BR, Denio LS and Drake ME (1990) Comparison of a non-instrumented immunoassay for carbamazepine to high performance liquid chromatography and fluorescence polarization immunoassay. *Epilepsia* **37**, 480–484.

Commission for the Control of Epilepsy and Its Consequences (1978) Plan for Nationwide Action on Epilepsy, Vol 1. DHEW Publication No. (NIH) 78–276. Washington, D.C.: U.S. Department of Health Education and Welfare.

Commission on Classification and Terminology of the International League Against Epilepsy (1981) Proposal for revised clinical and electroencephalographic classification of epileptic seizures. *Epilepsia* **22**, 489–501.

Commission on Classification and Terminology of the International League Against Epilepsy (1989) Proposal for Revised Classification of Epilepsies and Epileptic Syndromes. *Epilepsia* **30**, 389–399.

Commission on Pediatric Epilepsy of the International League Against Epilepsy (1992) Workshop on Infantile Spasms. *Epilepsia* **33**(1), 195.

Consensus Panel on Surgery for Epilepsy (1990) National Institutes of Health consensus development Conference statement: surgery for epilepsy. *JAMA* **264**, 729–733.

Covanis A, Gupta AK and Jeavons PM (1982) Sodium valproate: monotherapy and polytherapy. *Epilepsia* **23**, 693–720.

Cramer JA and Mattson RH (1979) Valproic acid: In vitro plasma protein binding and interaction with phenytoin. *Ther Drug Monit* **1**, 105–116.

Cramer JA and Russell ML (1988) Strategies to enhance adherence to a medical regimen. *Epilepsy Res* **1** (Suppl 1), 163–175.

Cranford RE, Leppik IE, Patrick B, Anderson CB and Kostick B (1979) Intravenous phenytoin in acute treatment of seizures. *Neurology* **29**, 1474–1479.

Currier RD, Kooi KA and Saidman J (1963) Prognosis of pure petit mal: a follow-up study. *Neurology* **13**, 959–967.

Dahllof G, Preber H, Eliasson S, Ryden H, Karsten J and Modeer T (1993) Periodontal condition of epileptic adults treated long-term with phenytoin or carbamazepine. *Epilepsia* **34**, 960–964.

Dallof G, Axio E and Modeer T (1991) Regression of phenytoin-induced gingival overgrowth after withdrawal of medication. *Swed Dent J* **15**, 139–143.

Daly DD (1975) Ictal clinical manifestations of complex partial seizures. In Penry, JK and Daly DD (Eds) *Advances in Neurology, Vol 11: Complex Partial Seizures and Their Treatment*. New York: Raven Press, pp. 57–83.

Daly D (1990) Epilepsy and Syncope. In Daly DD and Pedley TA (Eds) *Current Practice of Clinical Electroencephalography*. New York: Raven Press, pp. 269–334.

Dam M, Ekberg R, Loyning Y, Waltimo O and Jakobsen K (1989) A double-blind study comparing oxcarbazepine and carbamazepine in patients with newly diagnosed, previously untreated epilepsy. *Epilepsy Res* **3**, 70–76.

Dam M (1990) Children with epilepsy: the effect of seizures, syndromes, and etiological factors on cognitive functioning. *Epilepsia* **31** (Suppl 4), S26–S29.

Dana-Haeri J, Oxley J and Richens A (1982) Reduction of free testosterone by antiepileptic drugs. *Br Med J* **284**, 85–86.

Dawson GD (1947) Investigations on a patient subject to myoclonic seizures after sensory stimulation. *J Neurol, Neurosurg Psychiatry* **10**, 141–162.

Dean JC and Penry JK (1988) Carbamazepine/valproate therapy in 100 patients with partial seizures failing carbamazepine monotherapy: Long-term follow-up. *Epilepsia* **29**, 687.

Dean JC, Penry JK and Smith LD (1988) When carbamazepine monotherapy fails to control partial seizures. *Ann Neurol* **24**, 135.

Delgado-Escueta AV, Bacsal FE and Treiman DM (1981a) Complex partial seizures on closed-circuit television and EEG: A study of 691 attacks in 79 patients. *Ann Neurol* **11**, 292–300.

Delgado-Escueta AV, Mattson RH, King L, Goldensohn ES, Spiegel H, Madsen J, Crandall P, Dreifuss F and Porter RJ (1981b) The nature of aggression during epileptic seizures. *N Engl J Med* **305**, 711–716.

Delgado-Escueta AV, Wasterlain C, Treiman DM and Porter RJ (1982) Current concepts in neurology: Management of status epilepticus. *N Engl J Med* **306**, 1337–1340.

Delgado-Escueta AV and Enrile-Bascal FE (1984) Juvenile myoclonic epilepsy of Janz. *Neurology* **34**, 285–294.

Delgado-Escueta AV, Ward AA, Woodbury DM and Porter RJ (1986) New wave of research in the epilepsies. In Delgado-Escueta AV, Ward AA, Woodbury DM and Porter RJ (Eds) *Basic Mechanisms of the Epilepsies*. New York: Raven Press, pp. 3–55.

Delgado-Escueta AV, Greenberg DA, Treiman L., Liu A., Sparkes RS, Barbetti A, Park MS and Terasaki PI (1989) Mapping the gene for juvenile myoclonic epilepsy. *Epilepsia* **30**, S8–S18.

Delgado-Escueta AV, Swartz B, Chauvel P, Bancaud J, Walsh GO, Halgren E, Rich JR and Dwan P (1992) Clinical and CCTV-EEG evaluation in presurgical workup of temporal and frontal lobe epilepsies. In Theodore WH (Ed.) *Surgical Treatment of Epilepsy. Epilepsy Research Suppl 5*. Amsterdam: Elsevier, pp. 37–54.

Delgado-Escueta AV, Serratosa JM, Liu A, Weissbecker K, Medina MT, Gee M, Treiman LJ and Sparkes RS (1994) Progress in mapping human epilepsy genes. *Epilepsia* **35** (Suppl 1), S29–S40.

Desai BT, Riley TL, Porter RJ and Penry JK (1978) Active noncompliance as a cause of uncontrolled seizures. *Epilepsia* **19**, 447–452.

Desai BT, Porter RJ and Penry JK (1982) Psychogenic seizures: A study of 42 attacks in six patients, with intensive monitoring. *Arch Neurol* **39**, 202–209.

Devinsky O, Sato S, Kufta CV, Ito B, Rose DF, Theodore WH and Porter RJ (1989a) Electroencephalographic studies of simple partial seizures with subdural electrode recordings. *Neurology* **39**, 527–534.

Devinsky O, Putnam F, Grafman J, Bromfield E and Theodore WH (1989b) Dissociative states and epilepsy. *Neurology* **39**, 835–841.

Devinsky O (1991) Interictal behavioral changes in epilepsy. In Devinsky O and Theodore WH (Eds) *Epilepsy and Behavior*. New York: Wiley-Liss, pp. 1–22.

Devinsky O and Theodore WH (1991) *Epilepsy and Behavior*. New York: Wiley-Liss.

Devinsky O, Kothari M, Rubin R, Mercandetti R and Luciano D (1992) Felbamate for absence seizures. *Epilepsia* **33** (Suppl 3), 84.

REFERENCES

Devinsky O (1993) Clinical uses of the quality of life in epilepsy inventory. *Epilepsia* **34** (Suppl 4), 39–44.

Devinsky O and Cramer JA (1993) Introduction: quality of life in epilepsy. *Epilepsia* **34** (Suppl 4), 1–3.

Dieterich E, Baier WK, Doose H, Tuxhorn I and Fichsel H (1985a) Long-term followup of childhood epilepsy with absences. 1. Epilepsy with absences at onset. *Neuropediatrics* **16**, 149–154.

Dieterich E, Doose H, Baier WK and Fichsel H (1985b) Long term followup of childhood epilepsy with absences. 2. Absence epilepsy with initial grand mal. *Neuropediatrics* **16**, 155–158.

Dinesen H, Gram L, Anderson T and Dam M (1984) Weight gain during treatment with valproate. *Acta Neurol Scand* **70**, 65–69.

Dodrill CB, Batzel LW, Queisser HR and Temkin NR (1980) An objective method for the assessment of psychological and social problems among epileptics. *Epilepsia* **21**, 123–136.

Dodrill CB (1986) Correlates of generalized tonic-clonic seizures with intellectual, neuropsychological, emotional, and social function in patients with epilepsy. *Epilepsia* **27**, 399–411.

Dodrill CB, Wilkus RJ, Ojemann GA *et al.* (1986) Multidisciplinary prediction of relief from cortical resection surgery. *Ann Neurol* **20**, 2–12.

Dodrill CB (1987) Commentary: Psychological evaluation. In Engel JP (Ed.) *Surgical Treatment of the Epilepsies.* New York: Raven Press, pp. 197–201.

Dodrill CB and Troupin AS (1991) Neuropsychological effects of carbamazepine and phenytoin: a reanalysis. *Neurology* **41**, 141–143.

Dodson WE and Tasch V (1981) Pharmacology of valproic acid in children with severe epilepsy: clearance and hepatotoxicity. *Neurology* **31**, 1047–1050.

Dohrmann ML and Cheitlin MD (1986) Cardiogenic syncope: Seizure versus syncope. *Neurologic Clinics,* **4**, 549–562.

Dooley JM, Camfield PR, Camfield CS, Gordon KE and Fraser AD (1993) The use of antiepileptic drug levels in children: a survey of Canadian pediatric neurologists. *Can J Neurol Sci* **20**, 217–221.

Dowse R and Futter WT (1991) Outpatient compliance with theophylline and phenytoin therapy. *S Afr Med J* **80**, 550–553.

Dreifuss FE (1982) Ethosuximide: Toxicity. In Woodbury DM, Penry JK and Pippenger CE (Eds) *Antiepileptic Drugs* (second edition). New York: Raven Press, pp. 647–653.

Dreifuss FE and Sato S (1982) Benzodiazepines: Clonazepam. In Woodbury DM, Penry JK and Pippenger CE (Eds) *Antiepileptic Drugs* (second edition). New York: Raven Press, pp. 737–752.

Dreifuss F, Farwell J, Holmes G, Joseph C, Lockman L, Madsen JA, Minarcik CJ, Rothner AD and Shewmon DA (1986) Infantile spasms: Comparative trial of nitrazepam and corticotropin. *Archives of Neurology* **43**, 1107–1110.

Dreifuss FE (1987) Goals of surgery for epilepsy. In Engel JP (Ed.) *Surgical Treatment of the Epilepsies.* New York: Raven Press, pp. 31–50.

Dreifuss FE, Santilli N, Langer DH, Sweeney KP, Moline KA and Menander KB (1987) Valproic acid hepatic fatalities: A retrospective review. *Neurology* **37**, 379–385.

Dreifuss FE (1989) Valproate: toxicity. In Levy RH, Dreifuss FE, Mattson RH, Meldrum B, Penry JK (Eds) *Antiepileptic Drugs.* New York: Raven Press, pp. 643–652.

Dreifuss FE, Langer DH, Moline KA and Maxwell JE (1989) Valproic acid hepatic fatalities. II. US experience since 1984. *Neurology* **39**, 201–207.

Dreifuss FE (1990) Cognitive function: victim of disease or hostage to treatment? *Epilepsia* **33** (Suppl 1), 7–12.

Duchowney MS, Resnick TJ, Deray MJ and Alvarez LA (1988) Video EEG diagnosis of repetitive behavior in early childhood and its relationship to seizures. *Pediatric Neurology* **4**, 162–164.

Dulac O and Schlumberger E (1993) Treatment of West syndrome. In Wyllie E (Ed.) *The Treatment of Epilepsy: Principles and Practice*. Philadelphia: Lea and Febiger, pp. 595–603.

Duncan JS, Shorvon SD and Trimble MR (1990) Discontinuation of phenytoin, carbamazepine, and valproate in patients with active epilepsy. *Epilepsia* **31**, 324–333.

Dyken ME and Rodnitzky RL (1992) Periodic, aperiodic, and rhythmic motor disorders of sleep. *Neurology* **42** (Suppl 6), 68–74.

Eadie MJ, Tyrer JH, Bochner F and Hooper WD (1976) The elimination of phenytoin in man. *Clin Exp Pharmacol Physiol* **3**, 217–224.

Eadie MJ (1991) Formation of active metabolites of anticonvulsant drugs: a review of their pharmacokinetic and therapeutic significance. *Clin Pharmacokinet* **21**, 27–41.

Earnest MP, Thomas GE, Eden RA and Hossack KF (1992) The sudden unexplained death syndrome in epilepsy: demographic, clinical, and postmortem features. *Epilepsia* **33**, 310–316.

Efron R (1961) Post-epileptic paralysis: Theoretical critique and report of a case. *Brain* **84**, 381–394.

Eichelbaum M, Bertilsson L, Lund L, Palmer L and Sjoqvist F (1976) Plasma levels of carbamazepine and carbamazepine 10, 11-epoxide during treatment of epilepsy. *Eur J Clin Pharmacol* **9**, 417–421.

Ellison PH, Horn JL, Franklin S and Jones MG (1986) The results of checking a scoring system for neonatal seizures. *Neuropediatrics* **17**, 152–157.

Elster AD and Mirza W (1991) MR imaging in chronic partial epilepsy. Role of contrast enhancement. *AJNR* **12**, 165–70.

Elwes RDC, Chesterman P and Reynolds EH (1985) Prognosis after a first untreated tonic–clonic seizure. *Lancet* **2**, 752–753.

Emerson R, D'Souza BJ, Vining EP, Holden KR, Mellits ED and Freeman JM (1981) Stopping medication in children with epilepsy: Predictors of outcome. *N Engl J Med* **304**, 1125–1129.

Engel J Jr (1989) *Epilepsy*. Philadelphia: F.A. Davis. 536 pp.

Engel J Jr, Ludwig BI and Fetell M (1978) Prolonged partial complex status epilepticus: EEG and behavioral observations. *Neurology* **28**, 863–869.

Engel J Jr, Rausch R, Leib JP, Kuhl DE and Crandall PH (1981) Correlation of criteria used for localizing epileptic foci in patients considered for surgical therapy of epilepsy. *Ann Neurol* **9**, 215–224.

Engel J Jr, Kuhl DE, Phelps ME and Crandall PH (1982a) Comparative localization of epileptic foci in partial epilepsy by PCT and EEG. *Ann Neurol* **12**, 529–537.

Engel J Jr, Kuhl DE, Phelps ME and Mazziotta JC (1982b) Interictal cerebral glucose metabolism in partial epilepsy and its relation to EEG changes. *Ann Neurol* **12**, 510–517.

Engel J Jr, Henry T, Risinger MW, Mazziotta JC, Sutherling WN, Levesque MF and Phelps ME (1990) Presurgical evaluation for epilepsy: relative contributions of chronic depth-electrode recordings versus FDG-PET and scalp-sphenoidal ictal EEG. *Neurology* **40**, 1670–1677.

Escueta AV, Kunze U, Waddell G, Boxley J and Nadel A (1977) Lapse of consciousness and automatisms in temporal lobe epilepsy: A videotape analysis. *Neurology* **27**, 144–155.

Fakhoury T, Abou-Khalil B and Newman K (1993) Psychogenic seizures in old age: a case report. *Epilepsia* **34**, 1049–1051.

Farrell K, Abbott FS, Orr JM, Applegarth DA, Jan JE and Wong PK (1986) Free and total serum valproate concentrations: Their relationship to seizure control, liver enzymes and plasma ammonia in children. *Can J Neurol Sci* **13**, 252–255.

Farrell K (1993a) Classifying epileptic syndromes: problems and a biological solution. *Neurology* **43** (Suppl 5), S8–S11.

Farrell, K (1993b) Secondary Generalized Epilepsy and Lennox–Gastaut syndrome. In Wyllie E (Ed.) *The Treatment of Epilepsy: Principles and Practice*. Philadelphia: Lea and Febiger, pp. 604–613.

Farwell J, Milstein J, Opheim K, Smith E and Glass S (1984) Adrenocorticotrophic hormone controls infantile spasms independently of cortisol stimulation. *Epilepsia* **25**, 605–608.

Farwell JR, Lee YJ, Hirtz DG, Sulzbacher SI, Ellenberg JH and Nelson KB (1990) Phenobarbital for febrile seizures – effects on intelligence and on seizure recurrence. *N Engl J Med* **322**, 364–369.

Fast DK, Jones BD, Kusalic M and Erickson M (1986) Effect of carbamazepine on neuroleptic levels and efficacy. *Am J Psychiatr* **143**, 117–118.

Faught E, Sachdeo RC, Remler MP *et al.* (1993) Felbamate monotherapy for partial-onset seizures: an active control trial. *Neurology* **43**, 688–692.

Fejerman N and Di Blasi AM (1987) Status epilepticus of benign partial epilepsies in children: Report of two cases. *Epilepsia* **28**, 351–355.

Fejerman N (1991) Myoclonies et epilepsies chez l'enfant. *Rev Neurol* **147**, 782–797.

Felbamate Study Group in the Lennox–Gastaut Syndrome (1993) Efficacy of felbamate in childhood epileptic encephalopathy (Lennox–Gastaut Syndrome). *N Engl J Med* **328**, 29–33.

Fenichel GM (1985) *Neonatal Neurology*. New York: Churchill Livingstone, 342 pp.

First Seizure Trial Group (1993) Randomized clinical trial on the efficacy of antiepileptic drugs in reducing the risk of relapse after a first unprovoked tonic–clonic seizure. *Neurology* **43**, 478–483.

Foot M and Wallace J (1991) Gabapentin. *Epilepsy Res* Suppl 3, 109–114.

Forster FM and Booker HE (1984) The epilepsies and convulsive disorders. In Baker AB and Baker LH (Eds) *Clinical Neurology*, Vol 3, Chapter 31. Hagerstown: Harper and Row.

Fraser RT, Gumnit RJ, Thorbecke R and Dobkin BH (1993) Psychosocial rehabilitation; a pre- and postoperative perspective. In Engel JP Jr (Ed) *Surgical Treatment of the Epilepsies* (second edition). New York: Raven Press, pp. 669–677.

French JA, Williamson PD, Thadani VM, Darcey TM, Mattson RH, Spencer SS and Spencer DD (1993) Characteristics of medial temporal lobe epilepsy: I. Results of history and physical examination. *Ann Neurol* **34**, 774–780.

Friis ML, Kristensen O, Boas J, Dalby M, Deth SH, Gram LMM, Pedersen B, Sabers A, Worm-Petersen J, Andersen D and Jensen PK (1993) Therapeutic experiences with 947 epileptic outpatients in oxcarbazepine treatment. *Acta Neurol Scand* **87**, 224–227.

Froscher W, Burr W, Penin H, Vohl J, Bulau P and Kreiten K (1985) Free level monitoring of carbamazepine and valproic acid: clinical significance. *Clin Neuropharmacol* **8**, 362–371.

Furman JMR, Crumrine PK and Reinmuth OM (1990) Epileptic nystagmus. *Ann Neurol* 27, 686–688.

Gastaut H, Roger J, Soulayrol R *et al.* (1966) Childhood epileptic encephalopathy with diffuse slow spike-waves (otherwise known as "petit mal variant") or Lennox syndrome. *Epilepsia* 7, 139–179.

Gastaut H (1970) Clinical and electroencephalographic classification of epileptic seizures. *Epilepsia* 11, 102–113.

Gastaut H and Broughton R (1972) *Epileptic Seizures: Clinical and Electrographic Features, Diagnosis and Treatment*. Springfield, Ill.: Charles C Thomas. 286 pp.

Gastaut H. (1973) *Dictionary of Epilepsy*. Geneva: World Health Organization, 75 pp.

Gastaut H (1983) Classification of status epilepticus. In Delgado-Escueta AV, Wasterlain CG, Treiman DM and Porter RJ (Eds) *Advances in Neurology, Vol. 34: Status Epilepticus – Mechanisms of Brain Damage and Treatment*. New York: Raven Press, pp. 15–35.

Gates JR, Ramani V, Whalen S and Loewenson R (1985) Ictal characteristics of pseudoseizures. *Archives of Neurology* 42, 1183–1187.

Gates JR, Rosenfeld WE, Maxwell RE and Lyons RE (1987) Response of multiple seizure types to corpus callosum section. *Epilepsia* 28, 28–34.

Gates JR and Erdahl P (1993) Classification of non-epileptic events. In Rowan JA and Gates JR (Eds) *Non-Epileptic Seizures*. Boston: Butterworth-Heinemann, pp. 21–30.

Genton P, Michellucci B, Tassinari CA and Roger JC (1990) The Ramsay-Hunt syndrome revisited: mediterranean myoclonus versus mitochrondrial encephalomyopathy with ragged red fibers and baltic myoclonus. *Acta Neurol Scand* 81, 8–15.

Gilman JT, Alvarez LA and Duchowny MD (1993) Carbamazepine toxicity resulting from generic substitution. *Neurology* 43, 2696–2697.

Gjedde A (1989) The emancipation of Miss Menton. *J Cereb Blood Flow Metab* 9, 243–246.

Glaze DG, Hrachovy RA, Frost JD, Kellaway P and Zion TE (1988) Prospective study of outcome of infants with infantile spasms treated during controlled studies of ACTH and prednisone. *Journal of Pediatrics* 112, 389–396.

Glazko AJ, Peterson FE, Smith TC, Dill WA and Chang T (1982) Phenytoin metabolism in patients with long and short plasma half-lives. *Therap Drug Monit* 4, 281–292.

Gloor P, Olivier A and Ives J (1980) Loss of consciousness in temporal lobe seizures: Observations obtained with stereotaxic depth electrode recordings and stimulations. In Canger R, Angeleri F and Penry JK (Eds) *Advances in Epileptology: XIth Epilepsy International Symposium*. New York: Raven Press, pp. 349–353.

Gloor P (1984) Electroencephalography and the role of intracerebral depth electrode recordings in the selection of patients for surgical treatment of epilepsy. In Porter RJ, Mattson RH, Ward AA Jr and Dam M (Eds) *Advances in Epileptology: The XVth Epilepsy International Symposium*. New York: Raven Press, pp. 433–437.

Goldberg MA (1982) Eterobarb: Absorption, distribution, biotransformation, and excretion. In Woodbury DM, Penry JK and Pippenger CE (Eds) *Antiepileptic Drugs* (second edition). New York: Raven Press, pp. 803–811.

Goldstein DS, Spanarkel M, Pitterman A, Toltzis R, Gratz E, Epstein S and Keiser HR (1982) Circulatory control mechanisms in vasodepressor syncope. *American Heart Journal* 104, 1071–1075.

Goodridge DMG and Shorvon SD (1983) Epilepsy in a population of 6000. *Br. Med J* 287, 641–647.

REFERENCES

Gotman J, Ives JR and Gloor P (Eds) (1985) *Long-term Monitoring in Epilepsy* (EEG Suppl No. 37). Amsterdam: Elsevier, 444 pp.

Gowers WR (1885) *Epilepsy and Other Chronic Convulsive Diseases: Their Causes, Symptoms & Treatment.* Reprint. New York: Dover Publications, 1964, 255 pp.

Gram L and Jensen PK (1989) Carbamazepine: toxicity. In Levy R, Mattson R, Meldrum B, Penry JK and Dreifuss FE (Eds) *Antiepileptic Drugs.* New York: Raven Press, pp. 555–565.

Gram L, Sabers A and Dulac O (1992) Treatment of pediatric epilepsies with y-vinyl GABA (vigabatrin). *Epilepsia* 33 (Suppl 5), S26–29.

Grant SM, Faulds D (1992) Oxcarbazepine. A review of its pharmacology and therapeutic potential in epilepsy, trigeminal neuralgia and affective disorders. *Drugs* 43, 873–888.

Grasby PM, Frith CD, Friston KJ, Bench C, Frackowiak RSJ and Dolan RJ (1993) Functional mapping of brain areas implicated in auditory-verbal memory function. *Brain* 116, 1–20.

Greenberg DA and Delgado-Escueta AV (1993) The chromosome 6p epilepsy locus: Exploring mode of inheritance and heterogeneity through linkage analysis. *Epilepsia* 34 (Suppl 3), S12–S18.

Gross-Tsur V and Shinnar S (1993) Convulsive Status Epilepticus in Children. *Epilepsia* 34 (Suppl 1), S12–S20.

Gugler R and Mueller C (1978) Plasma protein binding of valproic acid in health and disease. *Br J Clin Pharmacol* 5, 441–446.

Gumnit RJ (Ed.) and Sell MA (Assoc. Ed) (1981) *Epilepsy: A Handbook for Physicians* fourth edition. Minneapolis: University of Minnesota Comprehensive Epilepsy Program, 64 pp.

Gumnit RJ (1993a) Psychogenic seizures. In Wyllie E (Ed.) *The Treatment of Epilepsy.* Philadelphia: Lea and Febiger, pp. 692–696.

Gumnit RJ (1993b) Inpatient multidisciplinary management of non- epileptic seizures. In Rowan JA and Gates JR (Eds) *Non-Epileptic Seizures.* Boston: Butterworth-Heinemann, pp. 269–274.

Haerer AF and Grace JB (1969) Studies of anticonvulsant levels in epileptics. 1. Serum diphenylhydantoin concentrations in a group of medically indigent outpatients. *Acta Neurol Scand* 45, 18–31.

Haidukewych D and Rodin EA (1985) Effect of phenothiazines on serum antiepileptic drug concentrations in psychiatric patients with seizure disorders. *Therap Drug Monit* 7, 401–404.

Hajek M, Antonini A, Leenders KL and Wieser HG (1993) Mesiobasal versus lateral temporal lobe epilepsy: metabolic differences in the temporal lobe shown by interictal 18F-FDG positron emission tomography. *Neurology* 43(1), 79–86.

Hallett M (1985) Myoclonus and epilepsy. *Epilepsia* 26 (Suppl 1), S67–77.

Halliday AM (1967) The clinical incidence of myoclonus. In Williams D (Ed.) *Modern Trends in Neurology,* Vol 4. London: Butterworths, pp. 69–105.

Hammond EJ, Ballinger WE, Lu L, Wilder BJ, Uthman BM and Reid SA (1992) Absence of cortical white matter changes in three patients undergoing long-term vigabatrin therapy. *Epilepsy Res* 12, 261–265.

Hanson JW and Smith DW (1975) The fetal hydantoin syndrome. *Journal of Pediatrics* 87, 285–290.

Hanson JW and Buehler BA (1982) Fetal hydantoin syndrome: Current status. *Journal of Pediatrics* 101, 816–818.

Harper M and Roth M (1962) Temporal lobe epilepsy and the phobic anxiety-depersonalization syndrome. Part I: A comparative study. *Comprehensive Psychiatry* 3, 129–151.

Hart RG and Easton JD (1982) Carbamazepine and hematological monitoring. *Ann Neurol* 11, 309–312.

Hauser WA and Kurland LT (1975) The epidemiology of epilepsy in Rochester, Minnesota, 1935 through 1967. *Epilepsia* 16, 1–66.

Hauser WA, Annegers JF and Elveback LR (1980) Mortality in patients with epilepsy. *Epilepsia* 21, 399–412.

Hauser WA, Anderson VE, Loewenson RB and McRoberts SM (1982) Seizure recurrence after a first unprovoked seizure. *N Engl J Med* 307, 522–528.

Hauser WA and Hesdorffer DC (1990) Risk Factors. In Hauser WA and Hesdorffer DC (Eds) *Epilepsy: Frequency, Causes, and Consequences.* New York: Demos, pp. 53–92.

Hauser WA and Hesdorffer DC (1990) Epilepsy: frequency, causes, and consequences. New York: Demos Publications, pp. 197–244.

Henrichs TF, Tucker DM, Farha J and Novelly RA (1988) MMPI indices in the identification of patients evidencing pseudoseizures. *Epilepsia* 29, 184–187.

Henricksen O and Johannessen SI (1982) Clinical and pharmacokinetic observations on sodium valproate. A five year follow-up study in 100 children with epilepsy. *Acta Neurol Scand* 65, 504–523.

Henry TR, Leppik IE, Gumnit RJ and Jacobs M (1988) Progressive myclonus epilepsy treated with zonisamide. *Neurology* 38, 928–931.

Hermann BP, Wyler AR, Richey ET and Rea JM (1987) Memory function and verbal learning ability in patients with complex partial seizures of temporal lobe origin. *Epilepsia* 28, 547–554.

Herranz JL, Armijo JA and Arteaga R (1988) Clinical side effects of phenobarbital, primidone, phenytoin, carbamazepine, and valproate during monotherapy in children. *Epilepsia* 29, 794–804.

Hirtz DG and Nelson KB (1985) Cognitive effects of antiepileptic drugs. In Pedley TA, Meldrum BS (Eds) *Recent Advances in Epilepsy 2.* Edinburgh: Churchill Livingstone, pp. 161–182.

Hirtz DG (1989) Generalized tonic–clonic and febrile seizures. *Ped Clin NA* 36, 375–383.

Hoefnagels WAJ, Padberg GW, Overweg J and Roos RAC (1992) Syncope or seizure? A matter of opinion. *Clinical Neurology and Neurosurgery* 94, 153–156.

Hoeppener RJ, Kuyer A, Meijer JWA and Hulsman J (1980) Correlation between daily fluctuations of carbamazepine serum levels and intermittent side effects. *Epilepsia* 21, 341–350.

Holmes GL, McKeever M and Adamson M (1987) Absence seizures in children: Clinical and electroencephalographic features. *Ann Neurol* 21, 268–273.

Holmes GL (1992) Rolandic epilepsy: clinical and electroencephalographic features. *Epilepsy Research* Suppl 6, 29–43.

Howe JG and Gibson JD (1982) Uncinate seizures and tumors: A myth reexamined. *Ann Neurol* 12, 227.

Hrachovy RA (1982) Infantile spasms. In *Classification of the Epilepsies: Age Related Syndromic Seizure Types. State of the Science in EEG and Epilepsy.* Annual Meeting of the American EEG Society and the American Epilepsy Society, Phoenix, 1982.

Hrachovy RA, Frost JD, Kellaway P and Zion TE (1983) Double-blind study of ACTH vs prednisone therapy in infantile spasms. *Journal of Pediatrics* 103, 641–645.

Hrachovy RA, Frost JD, Gospe SM and Glaze DG (1987) Infantile spasms following near-drowning: A report of two cases. *Epilepsia* 28, 45–48.

Hugg JW, Laxer KD, Matson GB, Maudsley AA and Weiner MW (1993) Neuron loss localizes human temporal lobe epilepsy by in vivo proton magnetic resonance spectroscopic imaging. *Ann Neurol* 34, 788–794.

Imaizumi T, Izumi T and Fukuyama Y (1992) A comparative clinical and pharmacokinetic study of a new slow-release versus conventional preparation of valproic acid in children with intractable epilepsy. *Brain Dev* 14, 304–308.

Isojarvi JI, Pakarinen AJ and Myllyla VV (1992) Thyroid function with antiepileptic drugs. *Epilepsia* 33, 142–148.

Isojarvi JI, Pakarinen AJ and Myllyla VV (1993) Serum lipid levels during carbamazepine medication: a prospective study. *Arch Neurol* 50, 590–593.

Jabbari B, Bryan GE, Marsh EE and Gunderson CH (1985) Incidence of seizures with tricyclic and tetracyclic antidepressants. *Arch Neurol* 42, 480–481.

Jack CR, Sharbrough FW, Twomey CK *et al.* (1990) Temporal lobe seizure lateralization with MR-based volume measurements of the hippocampal formation. *Radiology* 175, 423–429.

Jack CR, Sharbrough FW, Cascino GD *et al.* (1992) Magnetic resonance image-based hippocampal volumetry: correlation with outcome after temporal lobectomy. *Ann Neurol* 31, 138–146.

Jackson GD, Berkovic SF, Tress BM, *et al.* (1990) Hippocampal sclerosis can be reliably detected by magnetic resonance imaging. *Neurology* 40, 1869–1876.

Jacoby A, Johnson A and Chadwick D (1992) Psychosocial outcomes of antiepileptic drug discontinuation. *Epilepsia* 33, 1123–1131.

Janz D and Christian W (1957) Impulsiv-Petit mal. *Deutsche Zeitschrift fur Nervenheilkunde* 176, 346–386.

Janz D and Beck-Mannagetta G (1981) Abnormalities of delivery, gestation, and postnatal period in the offspring of epileptic parents: Retrospective study. *Epilepsia* 22, 373.

Janz D (1983) Etiology of convulsive status epilepticus. In Delgado-Escueta AV, Wasterlain CG, Treiman DM and Porter RJ (Eds) *Advances in Neurology, Vol 34: Status Epilepticus – Mechanisms of Brain Damage and Treatment*. New York: Raven Press, pp. 47–54.

Janz D (1985) Epilepsy with impulsive petit mal (juvenile myoclonic epilepsy). *Acta Neurol Scand* 72, 449–459.

Jayaker P, Duchowny M, Resnick T and Alvarez L (1992) Ictal head deviation: lateralizing significance of the pattern of head movement. *Neurology* 42, 1989–1992.

Jeavons PM (1977) Nosological problems of myoclonic epilepsies in childhood and adolescence. *Developmental Medicine and Child Neurology* 19, 3–8.

Jennum P, Friberg L, Fuglsang-Frederiksen A and Dam M (1994) Speech localization using repetitive transcranial magnetic stimulation. *Neurology* 44, 269–273.

Jolley ME, Stroupe SD, Schwenzer KS, Wang CJ, Lusteffes M, Hill HD, Popelka SR, Holen JT and Kelso DM (1981) Fluorescence polarization immunoassay III. An automated system for therapeutic drug determination. *Clin Chem* 27, 1575–1579.

Jones-Gotman M (1987) Commentary: psychological evaluation – testing hippocampal function. In Engel JP Jr (Ed.) *Surgical Treatment of the Epilepsies*. New York: Raven Press, pp. 161–172.

Jones-Gotman M (1991) Localization of lesions by neuropsychological testing. *Epilepsia* 32 (Suppl 5), S41–S52.

Jusko WJ (1976) Bioavailability and disposition kinetics of phenytoin in man. In Kellaway P and Petersen I (Eds) *Quantitative Analytic Studies In Epilepsy*. New York: Raven Press, pp. 115–136.

Kalsbeek WD, McLaurin RL, Harris BSH and Miller JD (1980) The national head and spinal cord injury survey: Major findings. *Journal of Neurosurgery* 53, S19–S31.

Kaneko S, Suzuki K, Sato T, Ogawa Y and Nowura Y (1981) The problems of antiepileptic medication in the neonatal period: Is breast feeding advisable? *Epilepsia* 22, 375.

Kaneko S, Otani K, Kondo T, Fukushima Y, Nakamura Y, Ogawa Y, Kan R, Takeda A, Nakane Y and Teranishi T (1992) Malformation in infants of mothers with epilepsy receiving antiepileptic drugs. *Neurology* 42 (Suppl 5), 68–74.

Kapetanovic IM, Kupferberg HJ, Porter RJ, Theodore W, Schulman E and Penry JK (1981) Mechanism of valproate-phenobarbital interaction in epileptic patients. *Clin Pharm Therap* 29, 480–486.

Keilson MJ, Hauser WA, Magrill JP and Goldman M (1987) ECG abnormalities in patients with epilepsy. *Neurology* 37, 1624–1626.

Kellaway P, Hrachovy RA, Frost JD and Zion T (1979) A precise characterization and quantification of infantile spasms. *Ann Neurol* 6, 214–218.

Kelly EC (1939) *John Hughlings Jackson*. Medical Classics, 3, 915.

Keranen T, Sillanpaa M and Reikkinen PJ (1988) Distribution of seizure types in an epileptic population. *Epilepsia* 29, 1–7.

Ketter TA, Malow BA, Flamini JR, White SR, Post RM and Theodore WH (1994) Anticonvulsant withdrawal-emergent psychopathology. *Neurology* 44, 55–61.

King DW, Gallagher BB, Murro AM and Campbell LR (1993) Convulsive non-epileptic seizures. In Rowan JA and Gates JR (Eds) *Non-Epileptic Seizures*. Boston: Butterworth-Heinemann, pp. 31–37.

Kinsman SL, Vining EPG, Quaskey SA, Mellits D and Freeman JM (1992) Efficacy of the ketogenic diet for intractable seizure disorders: review of 58 cases. *Epilepsia* 33, 1132–1136.

Klawans HL (1979) *Clin Neuropharmacol*, Vol 4. New York: Raven Press, 228 pp.

Koeppen D, Baruzzi A, Capozza M *et al.* (1987) Clobazam in therapy-resistant patients with partial epilepsy: a double-blind placebo-controlled crossover study. *Epilepsia* 28, 495–506.

Koskiniemi M, Donner M, Majuri H, Haltia M and Norio R (1974) Progressive myoclonus epilepsy: a clinical and histopathological study. *Acta Neurol Scand* 50, 307–332.

Krumholz A, Fisher RS and Weiss HD (1986) Persistent neurological deficits following complex partial status epilepticus (CPSE). *Epilepsia* 27, 614.

Kugelberg E and Widen L (1954) Epilepsia partialis continua. *EEG Clin Neurophysiol* 6, 503–506.

Kuks JBM, Cook MJ, Fish DR, Stevens JM and Shorvon SD (1993) Hippocampal sclerosis in epilepsy and childhood febrile seizures. *Lancet* 342, 1391–1394.

Kupferberg H (1978) Overview of antiepileptic drug analysis. In Pippenger CE, Penry JK, Kutt H (Eds) *Antiepileptic Drugs: Quantitative Analysis and Interpretation*. New York: Raven Press, pp. 9–15.

Kupferberg HJ, Yonekawa WD, Newmark ME, Porter RJ and Penry JK (1978) Measurement of mephenytoin and its demethylated metabolite, Nirvanol, by mass fragmentography in epileptic patients. Abstracts of the 7th International Congress of Pharmacology. Paris, p. 181.

Kupferberg HJ and Longacre-Shaw J (1979) Mephobarbital and phenobarbital plasma concentrations in epileptic patients treated with mephobarbital. *Ther Drug Monit* 1, 117–122.

REFERENCES

Kurlan R, Nutt JG, Woodward WR *et al.* (1988) Duodenal and gastric delivery of L-DOPA in Parkinsonism. *Ann Neurol* **23**, 589–595.

Kutt H, Winters W, Kokenge R and McDowell F (1964) Diphenylhydantoin metabolism, blood levels, and toxicity. *Arch Neurol* **11**, 642–648.

Kutt H, Solomon G, Wasterlain C, Peterson H, Louis S and Carruthers R (1975) Carbamazepine in difficult to control epileptic outpatients. *Acta Neurol Scand* **60** (Suppl), 27–32.

Kutt H (1989) Phenytoin: interactions with other drugs. In Levy R, Mattson RH, Meldrum B, Penry JK and Dreifuss FE (Eds) *Antiepileptic Drugs* (third edition). New York: Raven Press, pp. 215–232.

Kuzniecky R, de la Sayette V, Ethier R, Melanson D, Andermann F, Berkovic S, Robitaille Y, Olivier A, Peters T and Feindel W (1987) Magnetic resonance imaging in temporal lobe epilepsy: Pathologic correlations. *Ann Neurol* **22**, 341–347.

Kuzniecky R, Rubin ZK, Faught E and Morawetz R (1992) Antiepileptic drug treatment after temporal lobe epilepsy surgery: a randomized study comparing carbamazepine and polytherapy. *Epilepsia* **33**, 908–912.

Kuzniecky R, Elgavish GA, Hetherington HP, Evanochko WT and Pohost GM (1992) In vivo 31P magnetic resonance spectroscopy of human temporal lobe epilepsy. *Neurology* **42**, 1586–1590.

Kuzniecky R, Murro A, King D *et al.* (1993) Magnetic resonance imaging in childhood intractable partial epilepsies: pathologic correlations. *Neurology* **43**, 681–687.

Lacy JR and Penry JK (1976) *Infantile Spasms.* New York: Raven Press, 169 pp.

Lai C and Ziegler DK (1981) Syncope problem solved by continuous ambulatory simultaneous EEG/ECG recording. *Neurology* **31**, 1152–1154.

Larkin JG, Herrick AL, McGuire GM, Percy-Robb IW and Brodie MJ (1991) Antiepileptic drug monitoring at the epilepsy clinic: a prospective evaluation. *Epilepsia* **32**, 89–95.

Laxer KD, Mullooly JP and Howell B (1985) Prolactin changes after seizures classified by EEG monitoring. *Neurology* **35**, 31–35.

Lee BI, Markand ON, Siddiqui AR, Park HM, Mock B, Wellman HH, Worth RM and Edwards MK (1986) Single photon emission computed tomography (SPECT) brain imaging using N, N, N′-trimethyl-N′-(2 hydroxy-3-methyl-5-123I-iodobenzyl)-1,3-propanediamine 2 HCl (HIPDM): intractable complex partial seizures. *Neurology* **36**, 1471–1477.

Lee BI, Markand ON, Wellman HN, Siddiqui AR, Park, HM, Mock B, Worth RM, Edwards MK and Krepshaw J (1988) HIPDM-SPECT in patients with medically intractable complex partial seizures: ictal study. *Arch Neurol* **45**, 397–402.

Lefebvre EB, Haining RG and Labbe R (1972) Coarse facies, calvarial thickening and hyperphosphatasia associated with long-term anticonvulsant therapy. *N Eng J Med* **286**, 1301–1302.

LeGarda S, Maria BL, Matsuo F, Allen FH, Runge JW, Kugler AR and Marriott JC (1993) Safety, tolerance, and pharmacokinetics of fosphenyoin, a phenytoin prodrug, in status epilepticus. *Epilepsia* **34** (Suppl 6), 60.

Leiderman DB (1993) Gabapentin as add-on therapy for refractory partial epilepsy: results of five placebo-controlled trials. *Epilepsia* **35** (Suppl 5), S74–S76.

Lemieux L, Lester S and Fish D (1992) Multimodality imaging and intracranial EEG display for stereotactic surgery and planning in epilepsy. *EEG Clin Neurophysiol* **82**, 399–407.

Lencz T, McCarthy G, Bronen RA *et al.* (1992) Quantitative magnetic resonance imaging in temporal lobe epilepsy: relationship to neuropathology and neuropsychological function. *Ann Neurol* 31, 629–637.

Lenn NJ and Robertson M (1992) Clinical utility of unbound antiepileptic drug levels in the management of epilepsy. *Neurology* 42, 988–990.

Lennox WG (1960) *Epilepsy and Related Disorders*, Vol 1. Boston: Little, Brown. 574 pp.

Leppik IE, Derivan AT, Homan RW, Walker J, Ramsay RE and Patrick B (1983) Double-blind study of lorazepam and diazepam in status epilepticus. *JAMA* 249, 1452–1454.

Leppik I (1988) Compliance during treatment of epilepsy. *Epilepsia* 29 (Suppl 2), S79–S84.

Leppik IE, Boucher BA, Wilder BJ, Murthy VS, Watridge C, Graves NM, Rangel RJ, Rask CA and Turlapaty P (1990) Pharmacokinetics and safety of a phenytoin prodrug given IV or IM in patients. *Neurology* 40, 456–460.

Leppik IE, Dreifuss FE, Pledger GW *et al.* (1991) Felbamate for partial seizures; results of a controlled clinical trial. *Neurology* 41, 1785–1789.

Leppik IE (1992) Metabolism of antiepileptic medication: newborn to elderly. *Epilepsia* 33 (Suppl 4), S32–40.

Lerman P and Kivity S (1982) The efficacy of corticotropin in primary infantile spasms. *Journal of Pediatrics* 101, 294–296.

Lesser RP, Pippenger CE, Luders H and Dinner DS (1984) High dose monotherapy in treatment of intractable seizures. *Neurology* 34, 707–711.

Levy G (1993) A pharmacokinetic perspective on medicament noncompliance. *Clin Pharm Therap* 54, 242–244.

Levy M, Goodman MW, Van Dyne B and Summer HW (1981) Granulomatous hepatitis secondary to carbamazepine. *Ann Internal Med* 95, 64–65.

Lewis RJ, Yee L, Inkelis SH and Gilmore D (1993) Clinical predictors of post-traumatic seizures in children with head trauma. *Annals of Emergency Medicine* 22,1114–1118.

Liewendahl K, Majuri H and Helenius T (1978) Thyroid function tests in patients on long-term treatment with various anticonvulsant drugs. *Clin Endocrinol* 8, 185–191.

Lindhout D, Omtzigt JGC and Cornel MC (1992) Spectrum of neural-tube defects in 34 infants prenatally exposed to antiepileptic drugs. *Neurology* 42 (Suppl 5), 111–118.

Lindsay J, Ounstead C and Richards P (1979) Long-term outcome in children with temporal lobe seizures. 1: social outcome and childhood factors. *Devel Med Child Neurol* 21, 285–298.

Lindsay J, Glaser G, Richards P and Ounstead C (1984) Developmental aspects of focal epilepsies treated by neurosurgery. *Devel Med Child Neurol* 26, 574–587.

Lipman IJ (1993) Epilepsy and driving. *AES News* 2(2), 4–8.

Loiseau, P and Duche B (1989) Benign childhood epilepsy with centrotemporal spikes. *Cleveland Clinic Journal of Medicine* 56 (Suppl 1), 17–22.

Loiseau P, Pestre M, Dartigues JF, Commenges D, Barberger-Gateau C and Cohadon S (1983) Long-term prognosis in two forms of childhood epilepsy: typical absence seizures and epilepsy with rolandic (centrotemporal) EEG foci. *Ann Neurol* 13, 642–648.

Loiseau P, Duche B and Loiseau J (1991) Classification of epilepsies and epileptic syndromes in two different samples of patients. *Epilepsia* 32, 303–309.

Lombroso CT (1967) Sylvian seizures and midtemporal spike foci in children. *Arch Neurol* 17, 52–59.

Lombroso CT and Holmes GL (1993) Value of the EEG in neonatal seizures. *Journal of Epilepsy* 6, 39–70.

Lorenzo NY, Bromfield EB and Theodore WH (1988) Phenytoin and carbamazepine:

Combination versus single-drug therapy for intractable partial seizures. *Ann Neurol* 24, 136.

Loring DW, Murro AM, Lee GP *et al.* (1993) Wada memory testing and hippocampal volume measurements in the evaluation for temporal lobectomy. *Neurology* 43, 1789–1793.

Luders H, Awad I, Burgess R, Wyllie E and Van Ness P (1992) Subdural electrodes in the presurgical evaluation for surgery of epilepsy. In Theodore WH (Ed.) *Surgical Treatment of Epilepsy. Epilepsy Research Suppl 5*. Amsterdam: Elsevier, pp. 147–156.

Macphee GJA, Goldie C, Roulston D *et al.* (1986) Effect of carbamazepine of psychomotor performance in naive subjects. *Eur J Clin Pharmacol* 31, 195–199.

Malherbe C, Burrill KC, Levin SR, Karam JH and Forsham PH (1972) Effect of diphenylhydantoin on insulin secretion in man. *N Engl J Med* 286, 339–342.

Malow BA, Blaxton TA, Stertz B and Theodore WH (1993) Carbamazepine withdrawal: effects of taper rate on seizure frequency. *Neurology* 43, 2280–2284.

Marciani MG, Gotman J, Andermann F and Olivier A (1985) Patterns of seizure activation after withdrawal of antiepileptic medications. *Neurology* 35, 1537–1543.

Marks RC and Luchins DJ (1991) Antipsychotic medications and seizures. *Psychiatr Med* 9, 37–52.

Marsden CD, Hallet M and Fahn S (1982) The nosology and pathophysiology of myoclonus. In Marsden CD and Fahn S (Eds) *Neurology 2: Movement Disorders*. London: Butterworths, pp. 196–248.

Matricardi M, Brinciotti M and Benedetti P (1989) Outcome after discontinuation of antiepileptic drug therapy in children with epilepsy. *Epilepsia* 30, 582–589.

Matsuo F, Bergen D, Faught E *et al.* (1993) Placebo-controlled study of the efficacy and safety of lamotrigine in patients with partial seizures. *Neurology* 43, 2284–2291.

Matthews WB (1976) Paroxysmal symptoms in multiple sclerosis. *J Neurol Neurosurg Psychiat* 38, 617–623.

Mattson RH (1980) Value of intensive monitoring. In Wada JA and Penry JK (Eds) *Advances in Epileptology: 10th International Symposium*. New York: Raven Press, pp. 43–51.

Mattson RH and Cramer JA (1980) Valproic acid and ethosuximide interaction. *Ann Neurol* 7, 583–584.

Mattson RH, Cramer JA, Collins JF *et al.* (1985) Comparison of carbamazepine, phenobarbital, phenytoin, and primidone in partial and secondarily generalized tonic–clonic seizures. *N Engl J Med* 313, 145–151.

Mattson RH and Cramer JA (1989a) Phenobarbital: Toxicity. In Levy RH, Dreifuss FE, Mattson RH, Meldrum BS and Penry JK (Eds) *Antiepileptic Drugs*. New York: Raven Press, pp. 329–340.

Mattson RH and Cramer JA (1989b) Valproate: interactions with other drugs. In Levy R, Mattson R, Meldrum B, Penry JK and Dreifuss FE (Eds) *Antiepileptic Drugs*. New York: Raven Press, pp. 621–632.

Mattson RH, Cramer JA and McCutchen CB (1989) Barbiturate related connective tissue disorders. *Arch Intern Med* 149(4), 911–914.

Mattson RH, Cramer JA, Collins JF *et al.* (1992) A comparison of valproate with carbamazepine for the treatment of complex partial seizures and secondarily generalized seizures in adults. *N Engl J Med* 327, 765–771.

Matuzas W and Jack E (1991) The drug treatment of panic disorder. *Psychiatr Med* 9, 215–243.

May RB and Sunder TR (1993) Hematologic manifestations of long-term valproate therapy. *Epilepsia* **34**, 1098–1101.

Mayeux R, Brandt J, Rosen J and Benson DF (1980) Interictal language and memory impairment in temporal lobe epilepsy. *Neurology* **30**, 120–125.

Maynert EW (1972) Phenobarbital, mephobarbital, and metharbital: Biotransformation. In Woodbury DM, Penry JK and Schmidt RP (Eds) *Antiepileptic Drugs*. New York: Raven Press, pp. 311–317.

Maytal J, Novak GP and King KC (1991) Lorazepam in the treatment of refractory neonatal seizures. *Journal of Child Neurology* **6**, 319–323.

McCarthy G, Blamire AM, Rothman DL, Gruetter R and Shulman RG (1993) Echoplanar magnetic resonance imaging studies of frontal cortex activation during word generation in humans. *Proc Natl Acad Sci USA* **90**(11), 4952–4956.

McKee PJ, Blacklaw J, Bulter E, Gillham RA and Brodie MJ (1991) Monotherapy with conventional and controlled-release carbamazepine: double-blind, double-dummy comparison in epileptic patients. *Br J Clin Pharmacol* **32**, 99–104.

McKee PJ, Blacklaw J, Friel E, Thompson G, Gillham RA and Brodie MJ (1993) Adjuvant vigabatrin in refractory epilepsy: a ceiling to effective dosage in individual patients? *Epilepsia* **34**, 937–943.

Meador KJ, Loring DW, Huh K, Gallagher BB and King DW (1990) Comparative cognitive effects of anticonvulsants. *Neurology* **40**, 391–394.

Meador KJ, Loring DW, Abney OL, Allen ME, Moore EE, Zamrini EY and King DW (1993) Effects of carbamazepine and phenytoin on EEG and memory in healthy adults. *Epilepsia* **34**, 153–157.

Medical Research Council Antiepileptic Drug Withdrawal Study Group (1991) Randomized study of antiepileptic drug withdrawal in patients in remission. *Lancet* **337**, 1175–1180.

Meierkord H, Will B, Fish D and Shorvon S (1991) The clinical features and prognosis of pseudoseizures diagnosed using video-EEG telemetry. *Neurology* **41**, 1643–1646.

Mendez MF, Doss RC and Taylor JL (1993) Interictal violence in epilepsy: relationship to behavior and seizure variables. *The Journal of Nervous and Mental Disease* **181**, 566–569.

Menkes JH (1985) *Textbook of Child Neurology*. Philadelphia: Lea and Febiger, 827 pp.

Merlis JK (1970) Proposal for an international classification of the epilepsies. *Epilepsia* **11**, 114–119.

Merlis JK (1972) Treatment in relation to classification of the epilepsies. *Acta Neurologica Latinoamericana* **18**, 42–51.

Messenheimer J, Ramsay RE, Willmore LJ, Leroy RF, Zielinski JJ, Mattson R, Pellock JM, Valakas AM, Womble G and Risner M (1994) Lamotrigine therapy for partial seizures: a multicenter, placebo-controlled, double-blind crossover trial. *Epilepsia* **35**, 113–121.

Metrakos K and Metrakos JD (1961) Genetics of convulsive disorders: II. Genetic and electroencephalographic studies in centrencephalic epilepsy. *Neurology* **11**, 474–483.

Meyer FB, Marsh WR, Laws ER and Sharbrough FW (1986) Temporal lobectomy in children with epilepsy. *J Neurosurg* **64**, 371–376.

Mitchell WG and Chavez JM (1987) Carbamazepine versus phenobarbital for partial onset seizures in children. *Epilepsia* **28**, 56–60.

Mizrahi EM and Kellaway P (1987) Characterization and classification of neonatal seizures. *Neurology* **37**, 1837–1844.

REFERENCES

Modigh K (1987) Antidepressant drugs in anxiety disorders. *Acta Psychiatr. Scand* **76** (Suppl 335), 57–71.

Monaco A, Riccio A, Benna P, Covacich A, Durelli L, Fantin M, Furlan PM, Gilli M, Mutani R, Troni W, Gerna M and Morselli PL (1976) Further observations on carbamazepine plasma levels in epileptic patients. *Neurology* **26**, 936–943.

Monday K and Janovic J (1993) Psychogenic myoclonus. *Neurology* **43**, 394–352.

Montouris GD, Fenichel GM and McLain LW Jr (1979) The pregnant epileptic: A review and recommendations. *Arch Neurol* **36**, 601–603.

Morrell MJ, Sperling MR, Stecker M and Dichter MA (1994) Sexual dysfunction in partial epilepsy: a deficit in physiological arousal. *Neurology* **44**, 243–248.

Morris JC, Dodson WE, Hatlelid JM and Ferrendelli JA (1987) Phenytoin and carbamazepine, alone and in combination: Anticonvulsant and neurotoxic effects. *Neurology* **37**, 1111–1118.

Munari C and Bancaud J (1985) The role of stereo-electroencephalography (SEEG) in the evaluation of partial epileptic seizures. In Porter RJ and Morselli PL (Eds) *The Epilepsies*. London: Butterworths, pp. 267–306.

Nelson KB and Ellenberg JH (1976) Predictors of epilepsy in children who have experienced febrile seizures. *N Engl J Med* **295**, 1029–1033.

Nelson KB and Ellenberg JH (1981) The role of recurrences in determining outcome in children with febrile seizures. In Nelson KB and Ellenberg JH (Eds) *Febrile Seizures*. New York: Raven Press, pp. 19–25.

Newmark ME and Porter RJ (1982) Clinical research trends in the genetics of epilepsy. In Anderson VE, Hauser WA, Penry JK and Sing CF (Eds) *Genetic Basis of the Epilepsies*. New York: Raven Press, pp. 161–168.

Ney GC, Schaul N, Loughlin J, Rai K and Chandra V (1994) Thrombocytopenia in association with adjunctive felbamate use (letter). *Neurology* **44**, 980–981.

Niedermeyer E (1976) Immediate transition from a petit mal absence into a grand mal seizure: Case report. *European Neurology* **14**, 11–16.

Niedermeyer E (1993a) Epileptic Seizure Disorders. In Niedermeyer E (Ed.) *Electroencephalography: Basic Principles, Clinical Applications, and Related Fields* (third edition, Chapter 28). Williams and Wilkins, pp. 461–564.

Niedermeyer E (1993b) Nonepileptic Attacks. In Niedermeyer E and Lopes da Silva F (Eds) *Electroencephalography*. Baltimore: Williams and Wilkins, pp. 565–572.

Novelly R, Augustine E, Mattson RH *et al.* (1984) Selective memory improvement and impairment in temporal lobectomy for epilepsy. *Ann Neurol* **15**, 64–67.

Nuwer MR, Browne TR, Dodson WE *et al.* (1990) Generic substitutions for antiepileptic drugs. *Neurology* **40**, 1647–1651.

Ochs R, Gloor P, Quesney F, Ives J and Olivier A (1984) Does head turning during a seizure have lateralizing or localizing significance? *Neurology* **34**, 884–890.

Offringa M, Derksen-Lubsen G, Bossuyt PM and Lubsen J (1992) Seizure recurrence after a first febrile seizure: a multivariate approach. *Devel Med Child Neurol* **34**, 15–24.

Ojemann GA and Dodrill C (1985) Verbal memory deficits after left temporal lobectomy for epilepsy. *J Neurosurg* **62**, 101–107.

Ojemann GA (1987) Surgical therapy for medically intractable epilepsy. *J Neurosurg* **66**, 489–499.

Ojemann LM, Baugh-Bookman C and Dudley DL (1987) Effect of psychotropic medications on seizure control in patients with epilepsy. *Neurology* **37**, 1525–1527.

Oles KS, Penry JK, Smith LD, Anderson RL, Dean JC and Riela AV (1992) Therapeutic bioequivalency study of brand name versus generic carbamazepine. *Neurology* **42**, 1147–1153.

Oles KS and Gal P (1993) Bioequivalency revisited: Epitol versus Tegretol. *Neurology* **43**, 2435–2436.

Olivier A (1990) Extratemporal resections in the surgical treatment of epilepsy. In Spencer SS, Spencer DD (Eds) *Surgery for Epilepsy*. Cambridge, Mass.: Blackwell, pp. 150–167.

Olivier A (1992) Temporal resections in the surgical treatment of epilepsy. In Theodore WH (Ed.) *Surgical Treatment of Epilepsy*. *Epilepsy Research Suppl 5*. Amsterdam: Elsevier, pp. 147–156; pp. 175–189.

Oller-Daurella L (1974) The confusional states (absence status) *Acta Neurologica Belgica* **74**, 265–275.

Overweg J, Binnie CD, Oosting J and Rowan AJ (1987) Clinical and EEG prediction of seizure recurrence following antiepileptic drug withdrawal. *Epilepsy Res* **1**, 272–283.

Painter MJ, Pippenger C, Wasterlain C, Barmada M, Pitlick W, Carter G and Abern S (1981) Phenobarbital and phenytoin in neonatal seizures: Metabolism and tissue distribution. *Neurology* **31**, 1107–1112.

Painter MJ (1989) Phenobarbital: clinical use. In Levy RH, Dreifuss FE, Mattson RH, Meldrum BS and Penry JK (Eds) *Antiepileptic Drugs*. New York: Raven Press, pp. 329–340.

Palmer KJ and McTavish D (1993) Felbamate: a review of its pharmacodynamic and pharmacokinetic properties, and therapeutic efficacy in epilepsy. *Drugs* **45**, 1041–1065.

Pedley TA (1983) Differential diagnosis of episodic symptoms. *Epilepsia* **24** (Suppl 1), S31–S44.

Pelekanos J, Camfield P, Camfield C and Gordon K (1991) Allergic rash due to antiepileptic drugs: clinical features and management. *Epilepsia* **32**, 554–559.

Pellock JM (1987) Carbamazepine side effects in children and adults. *Epilepsia* **28** (Suppl 3), S64–S70.

Pellock JM (1993) The differential diagnosis of epilepsy: nonepileptic paroxysmal disorders. In Wyllie E (Ed.) *The Treatment of Epilepsy*. Philadelphia: Lea and Febiger, pp. 697–706.

Pellock JM, Rao C and Earl N (1993) Lamotrigine safety and efficacy update - US experience. *Epilepsia* **34** (Suppl 6), 42–43.

Penry JK and Dreifuss FE (1969) Automatisms associated with the absence of petit mal epilepsy. *Arch Neurol* **21**, 142–149.

Penry JK, Porter RJ and Dreifuss FE (1975) Simultaneous recording of absence seizures with video tape and electroencephalography: A study of 374 seizures in 48 patients. *Brain* **98**, 427–440.

Penry JK and Newmark ME (1979) The use of antiepileptic drugs. *Ann Internal Med* **90**, 207–218.

Penry JK, Dean JC and Riela AR (1989) Juvenile myoclonic epilepsy: long-term response to therapy. *Epilepsia* **30** (Suppl 4), S19–S23.

Peterson GM, Khoo BH and Von Witt RJ (1991) Clinical response in epilepsy in relation to total and free serum levels of phenytoin. *Ther Drug Monit* **13**, 415–419.

Petker MA and Morton DJ (1993) Comparison of the effectiveness of two oral phenytoin products and chronopharmacokinetics of phenytoin. *J Clin Pharm Ther* **18**, 213–217.

Piafsky KM (1980) Disease-induced changes in the plasma binding of basic drugs. *Clin Pharmacokinet* **5**, 246–262.

REFERENCES

Pies RW and Shader RI (1994) Approaches to the treatment of depression. In Shader RI (Ed.) *Manual of Psychiatric Therapeutics*. Boston: Little, Brown, pp. 217–246.

Pippenger CE, Paris-Kutt H, Penry JK and Daly DD (1977) Proficiency testing in determination of antiepileptic drugs. *J Analyt Toxicol* 1, 118–122.

Porro MG, Kupferberg HJ, Porter RJ, Theodore WH and Newmark ME (1982) Phenytoin: An inhibitor and inducer of primidone metabolism in an epileptic patient. *Br J Clin Pharmacol* 14, 294–297.

Porter RJ, Penry JK and Dreifuss FE (1973) Responsiveness at the onset of spike-wave bursts. *Electroencephalography and Clinical Neurophysiology* 34, 239–245.

Porter RJ (1980) Etiology and classification of epileptic seizures. In Robb P (Ed.) *Epilepsy Updated: Causes and Treatment*. Chicago: Year Book Medical Publishers, pp. 1–10.

Porter RJ and Penry JK (1980) Phenobarbital: Biopharmacology. In Glaser GH, Penry JK and Woodbury DM (Eds) *Advances in Neurology, Vol 27: Antiepileptic Drugs – Mechanisms of Action*. New York: Raven Press, pp. 493–500.

Porter RJ, Schulman EA and Penry JK (1980) Phenytoin monotherapy in intractable epilepsy. In Canger R, Angeleri F and Penry JK (Eds) *Advances in Epileptology: XIth Epilepsy International Symposium*. New York: Raven Press, pp. 419–422.

Porter RJ (1981) Pharmacokinetic basis of intermittent and chronic anticonvulsant drug therapy in febrile seizures. In Nelson KB and Ellenberg JH (Eds) *Febrile Seizures*. New York: Raven Press, pp. 107–118.

Porter RJ and Sato S (1982) Secondary generalization of epileptic seizures. In Akimoto H, Kazamatsuri H, Seino M and Ward AA Jr (Eds) *Advances in Epileptology: XIIIth Epilepsy International Symposium*. New York: Raven Press, pp. 47–48.

Porter RJ (1983) Intractable seizures. In Browne TR and Feldman RG (Eds) *Epilepsy: Diagnosis and Management*. Boston: Little, Brown, pp. 355–361.

Porter RJ and Penry JK (1983) Petit mal status. In Delgade-Escueta AV, Wasterlain CG, Treiman DM and Porter RJ (Eds) *Advances in Neurology, Vol 34: Status Epilepticus – Mechanisms of Brain Damage and Treatment*. New York: Raven Press, pp. 61–67.

Porter RJ (1986) Antiepileptic drugs: Efficacy and inadequacy. In Meldrum BS and Porter RJ (Eds) *New Anticonvulsant Drugs*. London: John Libbey, pp. 3–15.

Porter RJ and Theodore WH (1986) Nonsedative approaches to antiepileptic drug therapy. *Merritt Putnam Quarterly* 3, 3–15.

Porter RJ (1987) How to initiate and maintain carbamazepine therapy in children and adults. *Epilepsia* 28 (Suppl 3), S59–S63.

Porter RJ and Nadi NS (1987) Investigations into pharmacotherapy of the focal epilepsies. In Wieser HG, Speckman E-J and Engel J (Eds) *The Epileptic Focus*. London: John Libbey, pp. 175–191.

Porter RJ and Pitlock WH (1987) Antiepileptic drugs. In Katzung BG (Ed.) *Basic and Clinical Pharmacology* (third edition). Norwalk: Appleton and Lange, pp. 262–278.

Porter RJ (1989) How to use antiepileptic drugs. In Levy RH, Mattson RH, Meldrum BS, Penry JK and Driefuss FE (Eds) *Antiepileptic Drugs* (third edition). New York: Raven Press, pp. 117–131.

Porter RJ and Malone TE (Eds) (1992) Biomedical Research: Collaboration and Conflict of Interest. Baltimore: Johns Hopkins University Press. 230 pp.

Porter RJ (1993) The absence epilepsies. *Epilepsia* 34 (Suppl 3) S42–S48.

Porter RJ and Rogawski MA (1993) Potential antiepileptic drugs. In Wyllie E (Ed) *The Treatment of Epilepsy*. Philadelphia: Lea and Febiger, pp. 974–985.

Porter RJ and Sato S (1993) Prolonged EEG and video monitoring in the diagnosis of seizure disorders. In Niedermeyer E and Lopes da Silva F (Eds) *Electroencephalography*. Baltimore: Williams and Wilkins, pp. 729–738.

Powell G, Polkey C and McMillan T (1985) The new Maudsley series of temporal lobectomy. I: short-term cognitive effects. *Br J Clin Psychol* **24**, 109–124.

Privitera M (1993) Clinical rules for phenytoin dosing. *Ann Pharmacother* **27**, 1169–1173.

Purves SJ, Hashimoto SA and Tse KS (1988) Successful desensitization of patients with carbamazepine allergy. *Epilepsia* **29**, 654.

Purves SJ, Wada JA, Woodhurst WB *et al.* (1988) Results of anterior corpus callosum section in 24 patients with medically intractable seizures. *Neurology* **38**, 1194–1201.

Quesney LF, Constain M, Rasmussen T, Olivier A and Palmini A (1992) Presurgical EEG investigation in frontal lobe epilepsy. In Theodore WH (Ed.) *Surgical Treatment of Epilepsy. Epilepsy Research Suppl 5*. Amsterdam: Elsevier, pp. 55–70.

Radke RA, Hanson MW and Hoffman JM (1993) Temporal lobe hypometabolism on PET: predictor of seizure control after temporal lobectomy. *Neurology* **43**, 1088–1092.

Ramsay RE (1993a) Advances in the pharmacotherapy of epilepsy. *Epilepsia* **34** (Suppl 5), 9–16.

Ramsay RE (1993b) Treatment of status epilepticus. *Epilepsia* **34** (Suppl 1), S71–S81.

Ramsay RE (1994) Clinical efficacy and safety of gabapentin. *Neurology* **44** (Suppl 5), S23–S30.

Ramsay RE, Wilder BJ, Berger JR *et al.* (1983) A double-blind study comparing carbamazepine with phenytoin as initial seizure therapy in adults. *Neurology* **33**, 904–910.

Rasmussen T, Olszewski J and Lloyd-Smith D (1958) Focal seizures due to chronic localized encephalitis. *Neurology* **8**, 435–445.

Rasmussen T (1983) Characteristics of a pure culture of frontal lobe epilepsy. *Epilepsia* **24**, 482–493.

Rausch R and Crandall P (1982) Psychological status related to surgical control of epileptic seizures. *Epilepsia* **23**, 191–202.

Reinvang I, Bjarveit S, Johannessen SI, Hagen OP, Larsen S, Fagerthun H and Gjerstad L (1991) Cognitive function and time of day variation in serum carbamazepine concentration in epileptic patients treated with monotherapy. *Epilepsia* **32**, 116–121.

Reiser SJ (1978) Humanism and fact-finding in medicine. *N Engl J Med* **299**, 950–953.

Reunanen M, Heinonen EH, Nyman L and Anttlia M (1992) Comparative bioavailability of carbamazepine from two slow-release preparations. *Epilepsy Res* **11**, 61–66.

Reutens DC, Bye AM, Hopkins IJ, Danks A, Somerville E, Wlash J, Bleasel A, Ouvrier R, Mackenzie RA, Manson JI, Bladin PF and Berkovic, SF (1993) Corpus callosotomy for intractable epilepsy: seizure outcome and prognostic factors. *Epilepsia* **34**, 904–909.

Rey E, Pons G and Olive G (1992) Vigabatrin: clinical pharmacokinetics. *Clin Pharmacokinet* **23**, 267–278.

Reynolds EH (1989) Phenytoin: toxicity. In Levy R, Mattson R, Meldrum B, Penry JK and Dreifuss FE (Eds) *Antiepileptic Drugs* (third edition). New York: Raven Press, pp. 241–255.

Reynolds EH (1992) γ-vinyl GABA (vigabatrin): clinical experience in adult and adolescent patients with intractable epilepsy. *Epilepsia* **33** (Suppl 5), 30–35.

Rho JM, Donevan SD and Rogawski MA (1994) Mechanism of action of the anticonvulsant felbamate: opposing effects on NMDA and GABA-A receptors. *Ann Neurol* **35**, 229–234.

REFERENCES

Riikonen R (1982) A long-term follow-up study of 214 children with the syndrome of infantile spasms. *Neuropediatrics* **13**, 14–23.

Riley TL (1980) Lying About Epilepsy (Letter to the editor.) *N Engl J Med* **303**, 644.

Riley TL (1982) Syncope and hyperventilation. In Riley TL and Roy A (Eds) *Pseudoseizures*. Baltimore: Williams & Wilkins, pp. 34–61.

Riley TL and Roy A (1982) *Pseudoseizures*. Baltimore: Williams & Wilkins, pp. 231.

Riva R, Albani F, Cortelli P, Gobbi G, Perucca E and Baruzzi A (1983) Diurnal fluctuations in free and total plasma concentrations of valproic acid at steady state in epileptic patients. *Ther Drug Monit* S191–S196.

Robert E and Rosa F (1983) Valproate and birth defects. *Lancet* **2**, 1142.

Robertson MM (1986) Current status of the 1,4- and 1,5 benzodiazepines in the treatment of epilepsy: the place of clobazam. *Epilepsia* **27**, s27–s41.

Rocca WA, Sharbrough FM, Hauser WA, Annegers JF and Schoenberg BS (1987) Risk factors for complex partial epilepsy: a population-based case control study. *Ann Neurol* **21**, 22–31.

Rogawski MA and Porter RJ (1990) Antiepileptic drugs: pharmacological mechanisms and clinical efficacy with consideration of promising developmental stage compounds. *Pharmacol Rev* **42**, 223–286.

Rosa FW (1991) Spina bifida in infants of women treated with carbamazepine during pregnancy. *N Engl J Med* **324**, 674–677.

Rose AL and Lombroso CT (1970) Neonatal seizure states: A study of clinical, pathological, and electroencephalographic features in 137 full-term babies with a long-term follow-up. *Pediatrics* **45**, 404–425.

Rosman NP, Colton T, Labazzo J et al. (1993) A controlled trial of diazepam administered during febrile illnesses to prevent recurrence of febrile seizures. *N Engl J Med* **329**, 79–84.

Rowan AJ and Scott DF (1970) Major status epilepticus. *Acta Neurol Scand* **46**, 573–584.

Rowan AJ, Binnie CD, de Beer-Pawlikowski NKB, Goedhart DM, Gutter T, van der Geest P, Meinardi H and Meijer JWA (1979) Sodium valproate: Serial monitoring of EEG and serum levels. *Neurology* **29**, 1450–1459.

Rowan JA and Gates JR (1993) *Non-Epileptic Seizures*. Boston: Butterworth-Heinemann.

Rowe CC, Berkovic SF, Sia STB et al. (1989) Localization of epileptic foci with postictal single photon emission computed tomography. *Ann Neurol* **26**, 660–668.

Ryan R, Kempner K and Emlen AC (1980) The stigma of epilepsy as a self-concept. *Epilepsia* **21**, 433–445.

Sachdeo R, Kramer LD, Rosenberg A and Sachdeo S (1992) Felbamate monotherapy: controlled trial in patients with partial onset seizures. *Ann Neurol* **32**, 386–392.

Sachdeo RC, Murphy JV and Kamin M (1992) Felbamate in juvenile myoclonic epilepsy. *Epilepsia* **33** (Suppl 3), 118.

Sackellares JC, Siegal GJ, Abou-khalil BW et al. (1990) Differences between lateral and mesial temporal metabolism interictally in epilepsy of temporal lobe origin. *Neurology* **40**, 1420–1426.

Saint-Hilare JM, Gilbert M, Bouvier G and Barbeau A (1980) Epilepsy and aggression: Two cases with depth electrode studies. In Robb P (Ed.) *Epilepsy Updated: Causes and Treatment*. Chicago: Year Book Medical Publishers, pp. 145–176.

Sander JWAS, Trevisol-Bittencourt PC, Hart YM and Shorvon SD (1990) Evaluation of vigabatrin as an add-on drug in the management of severe epilepsy. *J Neurol Neurosurg Psychiatr* **53**, 1008–1010.

Sander JWAS, Hart YM, Trimble MR and Shorvon SD (1991) Vigabatrin and psychosis. *J Neurol Neurosurg Psychiatr* **54**, 435–439.

Sass KJ, Spencer DD, Spencer SS, Novelly RA, Williamson PD and Mattson RH (1988) Corpus callosotomy for epilepsy: Neurologic and neuropsychological outcome. *Neurology* **38**, 24–28.

Satischandra P, Lavine L, Theodore WH, Jabbari B, Dreifuss FE and Schoenberg BS (1987) Risk factors associated with intractable complex partial seizures. *Epilepsia* **28**, 617.

Sato S, White BG, Penry JK, Dreifuss FE, Sackellares JC and Kupferberg HJ (1982) Valproic acid versus ethosuximide in the treatment of absence seizures. *Neurology* **32**, 157–163.

Sato S, Dreifuss FE, Penry JK, Kirby DD and Palesch Y (1983) Long-term follow-up of absence seizures. *Neurology* **33**, 1590–1595.

Sato S, Long RL and Porter RJ (1985) Monitoring at the National Institute of Neurological and Communicative Disorders and Stroke. In Gotman J, Ives JR and Gloor P (Eds) *Long-term Monitoring in Epilepsy* (EEG Suppl No. 37). Amsterdam: Elsevier, pp. 415–422.

Schaumann BA, Annegers JF, Johnson SB, Moore KJ, Lubozynski MF and Salinsky MC (1994) Family history of seizures in posttraumatic and alcohol-associated seizure disorders. *Epilepsia* **35**, 48–52.

Schmidt D (1981) The effect of pregnancy on the natural history of epilepsy: Review of the literature. *Epilepsia* **22**, 365.

Schmidt D (1982) Two antiepileptic drugs for intractable epilepsy with complex partial seizures. *J Neurol Neurosurg Psychiatr* **45**, 1119–1124.

Schmidt D (1983) Reduction of two drug therapy in intractable epilepsy. *Epilepsia* **24**, 368–376.

Schmidt D, Tsai J-J and Janz D (1983) Generalized tonic–clonic seizures in patients with complex partial seizures: natural history and prognostic relevence. *Epilepsia* **24**, 43–48.

Schmidt D, Canger R, Cornaggia C, Avanzini G, Battino D, Cusi C, Beck-Mannagetta G, Koch S, Rating D and Janz, D (1984) Seizure frequency during pregnancy and puerperium: The role of noncompliance and sleep deprivation. In Porter RJ, Mattson RH, Ward AA and Dam M (Eds) *Advances in Epileptology: XVth Epilepsy International Symposium*. New York: Raven Press, pp. 221–225.

Schmidt D, Einicke I and Haenel F (1986) The influence of seizure type on the efficacy of plasma concentrations of phenytoin, phenobarbital, and carbamazepine. *Arch Neurol* **43**, 263–265.

Schmidt D, Jacob R, Loiseau P, Deisenhammer E, Klinger D, Despland A, Egli M, Bauer G, Stenzel E and Blankenhorn V (1993) Zonisamide for add-on treatment of refractory partial epilepsy: a European double-blind trial. *Epilepsy Res* **15**, 67–73.

Schmitz B and Wolf P (1991) Psychoses in epilepsy. In Devinsky O, Theodore WH (Eds) *Epilepsy and Behavior*. New York: Wiley-Liss, pp. 97–128.

Schottelius DD (1978) Homogeneous immunassay system (EMIT) for quantitation of antiepileptic drugs in biological fluids. In Pippenger CE, Penry JK and Kutt H (Eds) *Antiepileptic Drugs: Quantitative Analysis and Interpretation*. New York: Raven Press, pp. 95–108.

Schramm W, Annesley TM, Siegal GJ, Sackellares JC and Smith RH (1991) Measurement of phenytoin and carbamazepine in an ultrafiltrate of saliva. *Ther Drug Monit* **13**, 452–460.

REFERENCES

Schumacher GE, Barr JT, Browne TR, Collins JF, and the Veterans Administration Epilepsy Cooperative Study Group (1991) Test performance characteristics of the serum phenytoin concentration (SPC): the relationship between SPC and patient response. *Ther Drug Monit* **13**, 318–324.

Sennoune S, Mesdjian E, Bonneton J, Genton P, Dravet C and Roger D (1992) Interactions between clobazam and standard antiepileptic drugs in patients with epilepsy. *Ther Drug Monit* **14**, 269–274.

Serrano EE and Wilder BJ (1974) Intramuscular administration of diphenylhydantoin: Histologic follow-up studies. *Arch Neurol* **31**, 276–278.

Shafer SQ, Hauser WA, Annegers JF and Klass DW (1988) EEG and other early predictors of seizure remission: a community study. *Epilepsia* **29**, 590–600.

Sheehan DV (1982) Current concepts in psychiatry: Panic attacks and phobias. *N Engl J Med* **307**, 156–158.

Sherwin AL, Robb JP and Lechter M (1973) Improved control of epilepsy by monitoring plasma ethosuximide. *Archives of Neurology* **28**, 178–181.

Sherwin AL (1982) Ethosuximide: Relation of plasma concentration to seizure control. In Woodbury DM, Penry JK and Pippenger CE (Eds) *Antiepileptic Drugs* (second edition). New York: Raven Press, pp. 637–645.

Shibasaki H and Kuroiwa Y (1975) Electroencephalographic correlates of myoclonus. *EEG Clin Neurophysiol* **39**, 455–463.

Shibasaki H (1991) Motor phenomena of seizures. *Seminars in Neurology* **11**, 83–90.

Shields WD, Duchowny MS and Holmes GL (1993) Surgically remediable syndromes of infancy and early childhood. In Engel J Jr (Ed.) *Surgical Treatment of the Epilepsies.* New York: Raven Press, pp. 35–48.

Shinnar S, Vining EPG, Mellits ED, D'Souza BJ, Holden K, Baumgardner RA and Freeman JM (1985) Discontinuing antiepileptic medication in children with epilepsy after two years without seizures. *N Engl J Med* **313**, 976–980.

Shinnar S, Berg AT, Moshe SL, Kang H, O'Dell C, Alemany M, Goldensohn ES and Hauser WA (1994) Discontinuing antiepileptic drugs in children with epilepsy: a prospective study. *Ann Neurol* **35**, 534–545.

Shorvon SD and Reynolds EH (1982) Anticonvulsant peripheral neuropathy: a clinical and electrophysiological study of patients on single drug treatment with phenytoin, carbamazepine, or barbiturates. *J Neurol Neurosurg Psychiatr* **45**, 620–626.

Shorvon SD (1989) Clobazam. In Levy RH, Dreifuss FE, Mattson RH, Meldrum BS and Penry JK (Eds) *Antiepileptic Drugs.* New York: Raven Press, pp. 821–840.

Siemes H, Spohr HL, Michael Th and Nau H (1988) Therapy of infantile spasms with valproate: results of a prospective study. *Epilepsia* **29**, 553–560.

Siemes H, Nau H, Schultze K, Wittfoht W, Drews E, Penzien J and Seidel U (1993) Valproate (VPA) metabolites in various clinical conditions of probable VPA-associated hepatotoxicity. *Epilepsia* **34**, 332–346.

Simonsen N, Olsen IZ, Kuhl V, Lund M and Wendelboe J (1976) A comparative controlled study between carbamazepine and diphenylhydantoin in psychomotor epilepsy. *Epilepsia* **17**, 169–176.

Smith B and Dooley J (1993) Outcome of childhood epilepsy: a population-based study with a simple predictive scoring system for those treated with medication. *J Pediatr* **122**, 861–868.

Smith D, Baker G, Davies G, Dewey M and Chadwick DW (1993) Outcomes of add-on treatment with lamotrigine in partial epilepsy. *Epilepsia* **34**, 312–322.

Smith DB, Craft BR, Collins J, Mattson RH, Cramer JA and VA cooperative study group

118 (1986) Behavioral characteristics of epilepsy patients compared with normal controls. *Epilepsia* 27, 760–768.

Smith DB, Mattson RH, Cramer JA, Collins JF, Novelly RA and Craft B (1987) Results of a nationwide Veterans Administration cooperative study comparing the efficacy and toxicity of carbamazepine, phenobarbital, phenytoin, and primidone. *Epilepsia* 28 (Suppl 3), S50–S58.

Snead OC, Benton JW and Myers GJ (1983) ACTH and prednisone in childhood seizure disorders. *Neurology* 33, 966–970.

Sofijanov NJ (1982) Clinical evaluation and prognosis of childhood epilepsies. *Epilepsia* 23, 61–69.

Soryal I and Richens A (1992) Bioavailability and dissolution of proprietary and generic formulations of phenytoin. *J Neurol Neurosurg Psychiatr* 55, 688–691.

Specht U, Boenigk HE and Wolf P (1989) Discontinuation of clonazepam after long-term treatment. *Epilepsia* 30, 458–463.

Spencer SS (1981) Depth electroencephalography in selection of refractory patients for surgery. *Ann Neurol* 9, 207–214.

Spencer SS, Spencer DD, Williamson PD, Sass K, Novelly RA and Mattson RH (1988) Corpus callosotomy for epilepsy: seizure effects. *Neurology* 38, 19–24.

Spencer SS, Spencer DD, Williamson PD and Mattson RH (1990) Combined depth and subdural electrode investigation in uncontrolled epilepsy. *Neurology* 40, 74–79.

Spencer SS (1992) Depth electrodes. In Theodore WH (Ed.) *Surgical Treatment of Epilepsy. Epilepsy Research Suppl 5*. Amsterdam: Elsevier, pp. 135–146.

Spengler AF, Arrowsmith JB, Kilarski DJ, Buchanan C, Von Behren L and Graham DR (1988) Severe soft-tissue injury following intravenous infusion of phenytoin. *Arch Internal Med* 148, 1329–1333.

Sperling MR, Pritchard PB, Engel J, Daniel C and Sagel J (1986) Prolactin in partial epilepsy: an indicator of limbic seizures. *Ann Neurol* 20, 716–722.

Sperling MR, Wilson G, Engel J Jr, Babb TW, Phelps M and Bradley W (1986) Magnetic resonance imaging in intractable partial epilepsy: correlative studies. *Ann Neurol* 20, 57–62.

Sperling MR and O'Connor MJ (1989) Comparison of depth and subdural electrodes in recording temporal lobe seizures. *Neurology* 39, 1497–1504.

Spina E, Martines C, Fazio A, Trio R, Pisani F and Tomson T (1991) Effect of phenobarbital on the pharmacokinetics of carbamazepine 10,11 epoxide, an active metabolite of carbamazepine. *Ther Drug Monit* 13, 109–112.

Spitz MC (1991) Panic disorder in seizure patients: a diagnostic pitfall. *Epilepsia* 32, 33–38.

Stagno SJ (1993) Psychiatric aspects of epilepsy. In Wyllie E (Ed.) *The Treatment of Epilepsy*. Philadelphia: Lea & Febiger, pp. 1149–1162.

Stefan H, Pawlik G, Bocher-Schwarz HG, Biersack HJ, Burr W, Penin H and Heiss W-D (1987) Functional and morphological abnormalities in temporal lobe epilepsy: a comparison of interictal and ictal EEG, CT, MRI, SPECT, and PET. *J Neurol* 234, 377–384.

Stensrud PA and Palmer H (1964) Serum phenytoin determinations in epileptics. *Epilepsia* 5, 364–370.

Stevens H (1966) Paroxysmal choreoathetosis: a form of reflex epilepsy. *Arch Neurol* 14, 415–420.

Sugai K (1993) Seizures with clonazepam: discontinuation and suggestions for safe discontinuation rates in children. *Epilepsia* 34, 1089–1097.

REFERENCES

Sutton GG and Mayer RF (1974) Focal reflex myoclonus. *J Neurol Neurosurg Psychiatry* 37, 207–217.

Sutula TP, Sackellares JC, Miller JQ and Dreifuss FE (1981) Intensive monitoring in intractable epilepsy. *Neurology* 31, 243–247.

Swartz BE, Halgren E, Delgado-Escueta AV *et al.* (1989) Neuroimaging in patients with seizures of probable frontal origin. *Epilepsia* 30, 547–558.

Swartz BE, Tomiyasu U, Delgado-Escueta AV, Mandelkern M and Khonsari A (1992) Neuroimaging in temporal lobe epilepsy: test sensitivity and relationships to pathology and postoperative outcome. *Epilepsia* 33, 624–634.

Taylor DC (1993) Epilepsy as a chronic sickness. In Engel JP (Ed.) *Surgical Treatment of the Epilepsies.* New York: Raven Press, pp. 11–22.

Tatum WO, Sperling MR and Jacobstein JG (1991) Epileptic palatal myoclonus. *Neurology* 41, 1305–1306.

Taylor DC (1979) The components of sickness: diseases, illnesses, and predicaments. *Lancet* 2, 1008–1010.

Taylor J (Ed.) (1931) Selected Writings of John Hughlings Jackson, Vol 1: *On Epilepsy and Epileptiform Convulsions.* London: Hodder and Stoughton. Reprint 1958. New York: Basic Books.

Teare AJ (1980) True gestational epilepsy: A case report. *S Afr Med J* 57, 546–547.

Temkin O (1971) *The Falling Sickness.* Baltimore: Johns Hopkins, pp. 359–370.

Terrence CF, Rao GR and Perper JA (1981) Neurogenic pulmonary edema in unexpected, unexplained death of epileptic patients. *Ann Neurol* 9, 458–464.

Theodore WH and Porter RJ (1983a) Removal of sedative-hypnotic antiepileptic drugs from the regimens of patients with intractable epilepsy. *Ann Neurol* 13, 320–324.

Theodore WH and Porter RJ (1983b) Withdrawal of sedative-hypnotic antiepileptic drugs from outpatients. In Shorvon S and Birdwood G (Eds) *The Rational Prescription of Antiepileptic Drugs.* Berne: Hans Huber, pp. 95–99.

Theodore WH, Porter RJ and Penry JK (1983a) Complex partial seizures: Clinical characteristics and differential diagnosis. *Neurology* 33, 1115–1121.

Theodore WH, Schulman EA and Porter RJ (1983b) Intractable seizures: Long-term follow-up after prolonged inpatient treatment in an epilepsy unit. *Epilepsia* 24, 336–343.

Theodore WH, Newmark ME, Sato S, Brooks R, Patronas N, De La Paz R, DiChiro G, Kessler RM, Margolin R, Manning RG, Channing M and Porter RJ (1983c) 18F-fluorodeoxyglucose positron emission tomography in refractory complex partial seizures. *Ann Neurol* 14, 429–437.

Theodore WH, Qu Z-P, Tsay J-Y, Pitlick W and Porter RJ (1984a) Phenytoin: The pseudosteady-state phenomenon. *Clin Pharmacol Ther* 35, 822–825.

Theodore WH, Newmark ME, Desai BT *et al.* (1984b) Disposition of mephenytoin and its metabolite nirvanol in epileptic patients. Neurology 34, 1100–1102.

Theodore WH, Sato S and Porter RJ (1984c) Serial EEG in intractable epilepsy. *Neurology* 34, 863–867.

Theodore WH, Yu L, Price B, Yonekawa W, Porter RJ, Kapetanovic I, Moore H and Kupferberg H (1985a) The clinical value of free phenytoin levels. *Ann Neurol* 18, 90–93.

Theodore WH, Brooks R, Margolin R, Patronas N, Sato S, Porter RJ, Mansi L, Bairamian D and DiChiro G (1985b) Positron emission tomography in generalized seizures. *Neurology* 35, 684–690.

Theodore WH, DiChiro G, Margolin R, Fishbein D, Porter RJ and Brooks RA (1986a) Barbiturates reduce human cerebral glucose metabolism. *Neurology* 36, 60–64.

Theodore WH, Bairamian D, Newmark ME, DiChiro G, Porter RJ, Larson S and Fishbein D (1986b) Effect of phenytoin on human cerebral glucose metabolism. *J Cereb Blood Flow and Metab* **6**, 315–320.

Theodore WH, Dorwart R, Holmes M, Porter RJ and DiChiro G (1986c) Neuroimaging in refractory partial seizures: Comparison of PET, CT, and MRI. *Neurology* **36**, 750–759.

Theodore WH (1987) Should we measure free antiepileptic drug levels? *Clin Neuropharmacol* **10**, 26–37.

Theodore WH, Ito B, Devinsky O, Porter RJ and Jacobs G (1987a) Carbamazepine and cerebral glucose metabolism. *Neurology* **37**, 104.

Theodore WH, Porter RJ and Raubertas RF (1987b) Seizures during barbiturate withdrawal: Relation to blood level. *Ann Neurol* **22**, 644–647.

Theodore WH, Rose D, Patronas N, Sato S, Holmes M, Bairamian D, Porter RJ, DiChiro G, Larson S and Fishbein D (1987c) Cerebral glucose metabolism in the Lennox–Gastaut syndrome. *Ann Neurol* **21**, 14–21.

Theodore WH, Fishbein D, Deitz M and Baldwin P (1987d) Complex partial seizures: cerebellar metabolism. *Epilepsia* **28**, 319–323.

Theodore WH, Narang PK, Holmes MD, Reeves P and Nice FJ (1989a) Carbamazepine and its epoxide: Relation of plasma levels to toxicity and seizure control. *Ann Neurol* **25**, 194–196.

Theodore WH, Bromfield EB and Onorati L (1989b) The effect of carbamazepine on cerebral glucose metabolism. *Ann Neurol* **25**, 516–520.

Theodore WH (1990) Basic priniciples of clinical pharmacology. *Neurol Clin* **8**, 1–15.

Theodore WH, Katz D, Kufta C, Sato S, Patronas N, Smothers P and Bromfield E (1990) Pathology of temporal lobe foci: correlation with CT, MRI, and PET. *Neurology* **40**, 797–803.

Theodore WH, Raubertas R, Porter RJ *et al.* (1991) Felbamate: a clinical trial for complex partial seizures. *Epilepsia* **32**, 392–397.

Theodore WH (1992) Rational use of antiepileptic drug levels. *Pharmacol Ther* **54**, 297–305.

Theodore WH, Sato S, Kufta C, Balish MB, Bromfield EB and Leiderman DB (1992) Temporal lobectomy for uncontrolled seizures: the role of positron emission tomography. *Ann Neurol* **32**, 789–794.

Theodore WH, Jensen P and Kwan R (1994a). Felbamate: Clinical use. In Levy RH, Mattson RH and Meldrum BS (Eds) *Antiepileptic Drugs*. New York: Raven Press (in press).

Theodore WH, Porter RJ, Albert P, Kelley K, Bromfield EB, Devinsky O and Sato S (1994b). The secondary generalized tonic–clonic seizure: a video-tape analysis. *Neurology* **44**, 1403–1408.

Thomas JE, Reagan TJ and Klass DW (1977) Epilepsia partialis continua. A review of 32 cases. *Arch Neurol* **34**, 266–275.

Thomas KC, Hullin DA and Davis SJ (1991) Comparison of enzyme immunoassay and fluorescence polarization immunoassay as techniques for measuring anticonvulsant drugs on the same analytical instrument. *Ther Drug Monit* **13**, 172–176.

Thomason JM, Seymour RA and Rawlins MD (1992) Incidence and severity of phenytoin-induced gingival overgrowth in epileptic patients in general medical practice. *Community Dent Oral Epidemiol* **20**, 288–291.

Thurston JH, Thurston DL, Hixon BB and Keller AJ (1982) Prognosis in childhood epilepsy: additional follow-up of 148 children 15 to 23 years after withdrawal of anticonvulsant therapy. *N Engl J Med* **306**, 831–836.

Tomson, T (1984) Interdosage fluctuations in plasma carbamazepine concentration determine intermittent side effects. *Arch Neurol* **41**, 830–834.

Tomson T, Lindbom U, Ekqvist B and Sundqvist A (1994) Disposition of carbamazepine and phenytoin in pregnancy. *Epilepsia* **35**, 131–135.

Treiman DM and Delgado-Escueta AV (1983) Complex partial status epilepticus. In Delgado-Escueta AV, Wasterlain CG, Treiman DM and Porter RJ (Eds) *Advances in Neurology, Vol. 34: Status Epilepticus – Mechanisms of Brain Damage and Treatment*. New York: Raven Press, pp. 69–81.

Treiman DM (1986) Epilepsy and violence: Medical and legal issues. *Epilepsia* **27** (Suppl 2), S77–S104.

Treiman DM, Walton NY, Wickboldt C and DeGiorgio CM (1987) Predictable sequence of EEG changes during generalized convulsive status epilepticus in man and three experimental models of status epilepticus in the rat. *Neurology* **37** (Suppl 1), 244.

Treiman DM (1990) The role of benzodiazepines in the management of status epilepticus. *Neurology* **40** (Suppl 2), 32–42.

Treiman DM (1993) Generalized convulsive status epilepticus in the adult. *Epilepsia* **34** (Suppl 1), S2–S11.

Trennary MR, Jack CR, Ivnik RJ et al. (1993) MRI hippocampal volumes and memory function before and after temporal lobectomy. *Neurology* **43**, 1800–1805.

Triedman HM, Fishman RA and Yahr MD (1960) Determination of plasma and cerebrospinal fluid levels of dilantin in the human. *Trans Am Neurol Assoc* **85**, 166–170.

Trimble MR (1986) Pseudoseizures. In Porter RJ and Theodore WH (Eds) *Epilepsy*. Philadelphia: WB Saunders Neurologic Clinics, pp. 531–548.

Trimble MR and Robertson MM (1986) Clobazam. In Meldrum BS and Porter RJ (Eds) *New Anticonvulsant Drugs*. London: John Libbey, pp. 65–84.

Troupin AS, Ojemann LM and Dodrill CB (1976) Mephenytoin: A reappraisal. *Epilepsia* **17**, 403–414.

Troupin AS, Ojemann LM, Halpern L, Dodrill C, Wilkus R, Friel P and Feigl P (1977) Carbamazepine – a double-blind comparison with phenytoin. *Neurology* **27**, 511–519.

Tsai JJ, Lai ML, Yang YH and Huang JD (1992) Comparison on bioequivalence of four phenytoin preparations in patients with multiple dose treatment. *J Clin Pharmacol* **32**, 272–276.

Turnbull DM, Rawlins MD, Weightman D and Chadwick DW (1982) A comparison of phenytoin and valproate in previously untreated adult epileptic patients. *J Neurol Neurosur Psychiat* **45**, 55–59.

US Gabapentin Study Group (1993) Gabapentin as add-on therapy in refractory partial epilepsy: a double-blind, placebo-controlled, parallel group study. *Neurology* **43**, 2292–2298.

Uthman BM, Wilder BJ, Penry JK, Dean C, Ramsay RE, Reid SA, Hammond EJ, Tarver WB and Wernicke JF (1993) Treatment of epilepsy by stimulation of the vagus nerve. *Neurology* **43**, 1338–1345.

Van Allen MI, Fraser FC, Dallaire L, Allanson J, McLoed DR, Andermann E and Friedman JM (1993) Recommendations on the use of folic acid supplementation to prevent the recurrence of neural tube defects. *Canadian Medical Association Journal* **149**, 1239–1243.

Van Buren JM, Wood JH, Oakley J and Hambrecht F (1978) Preliminary evaluation of cerebellar stimulation by double-blind stimulation and biological criteria in the treatment of epilepsy. *J Neurosurg* 48, 407–416.

Van Buren J (1987) Complications of surgical procedures. In Engel JP (Ed.) *Surgical Treatment of the Epilepsies.* New York: Raven Press, pp. 465–475.

Van Woert MH and Rosenbaum D (1979) L-5-Hydroxytryptophan therapy in myoclonus. In Fahn S, Davis JN and Rowland LP (Eds) *Advances in Neurology, Vol 26: Cerebral Hypoxia and Its Consequences.* New York: Raven Press, pp. 107–122.

Vanderzant CW, Giordani B, Berent S, Dreifuss FE and Sackellares JC (1986) Personality of patients with pseudoseizures. *Neurology* 36, 664–668.

Vassella F, Pavlincova E, Schneider HJ, Rudin JH and Karbowski K (1973) Treatment of infantile spasms and Lennox–Gastaut syndrome with clonazepam. *Epilepsia* 14, 165–173.

Verity CM and Golding J (1991) Risk of epilepsy after febrile convulsions: a national cohort study. *Br Med J* 303, 1373–1376.

Verity CM, Ross EM and Golding J (1993) Outcome of childhood status epilepticus and lengthy febrile convulsions: finding of national cohort study. *BMJ* 307, 225–228.

Vickery BG (1993) A procedure for developing a quality of life measure for epilepsy surgery. *Epilepsia* 34 (Suppl 4), 22–27.

Victoroff JI, Benson DF, Grafton SI, Engel J Jr and Mazziotta JC (1994) Depression in complex partial seizures: electroencephalography and cerebral metabolic correlates. *Arch Neurol* 51, 155–163.

Villareal HJ, Wilder BJ, Willmore LJ, Baumann AW, Hammond EJ and Bruni J (1978) Effect of valproic acid on spike and wave discharges in patients with absence seizures. *Neurology* 28, 886–891.

Vining EPG, Mellits ED, Dorsen MM, Cataldo MF, Quaskey SA, Spielberg SP and Freeman JM (1987) Psychologic and behavioral effects of antiepileptic drugs in children: A double-blind comparison between phenobarbital and valproic acid. *Pediatrics* 80, 165–174.

Volpe JJ (1981) *Neurology of the Newborn.* Philadelphia: W.B. Saunders, 648pp.

Walton JN (1985) *Brain's Diseases of the Nervous System,* Ninth Edition. New York: Oxford University Press, 1701pp.

Walton NY (1993) Systemic effects of generalized convulsive status epilepticus. *Epilepsia* 34 (Suppl 1), S54–S58.

Wannamaker BB, Morton WA, Gross AJ and Saunders S (1980) Improvement in antiepileptic drug levels following reduction of intervals between clinic visits. *Epilepsia* 21, 155–162.

Wasterlain CG, Fujikawa DG, Penix L and Sankar R (1993) Pathophysiological mechanisms of brain damage after status epilepticus. *Epilepsia* 34 (suppl 1), s37–s53.

Waters CH, Belai Y, Gott PS, Shen P and DeGiorgio M (1994) Outcomes of pregnancy associated with antiepileptic drugs. *Arch Neurol* 51, 250–253.

Watson C, Andermann F, Gloor P, Jones-Gotman M, Peters T, Olivier A, Melanson D and Leroux G (1992) Anatomic basis of amygdaloid and hippocampal volume measurement by magnetic resonance imaging. *Neurology* 42, 1743–1750.

Weinberger J and Lusins J (1973) Simultaneous bilateral focal seizures without loss of consciousness. *Mt Sinai Medical Journal* 40, 693–696.

Welling PG (1984) Effects of gastrointestinal disease on drug absorption. In Benet LZ, Massoud N and Gambertoglio JG (Eds) *Pharmacokinetic Basis for Drug Treatment.* New York: Raven Press, pp. 63–76.

REFERENCES

Wieser H-G and Williamson PD (1993) Ictal semiology. In Engel JP Jr (Ed.) *Surgical Treatment of the Epilepsies* (second edition). New York: Raven Press, pp. 161–172.

Wieser H-G, Quesney L-F and Morris HH III (1993) Foramen Ovale and Peg electrodes. In Engel J Jr (Ed.) *Surgical Treatment of the Epilepsies*. New York: Raven Press, pp. 319–330.

Wilder BJ, Serrano EE and Ramsay RE (1973) Plasma diphenylhydantoin levels after after loading and maintenance doses. *Clin Pharm Therap* **14**, 798–801.

Wilder BJ and Ramsay RE (1976) Oral and intramuscular phenytoin. *Clin Pharm Therap* **19**, 360–364.

Wilder BJ and Buchanan RA (1981) Methsuximide for refractory complex partial seizures. *Neurology* **31**, 741–744.

Wilder BJ, Karas BJ, Hammond EJ and Perchalski RJ (1983) Twice daily dosing of valproate with divalproex. *Clin Pharm Therap* **34**, 501–504.

Williamson PD, Spencer DD, Spencer SS, Novelly RA and Mattson RH (1985) Complex partial seizures of frontal lobe origin. *Ann Neurol* **18**, 497–504.

Williamson PD (1992) Frontal Lobe Seizures: Problems of Diagnosis and Classification. In Chauvel P, Delgado-Escueta AV, Halgren E, and Bancaud J (Eds) *Frontal Lobe Seizures and Epilepsies*. New York. Raven Press.

Williamson PD (1993) Psychogenic non-epileptic seizures and frontal seizures: diagnostic considerations. In Rowan JA and Gates JR (Eds) *Non-Epileptic Seizures*. Boston: Butterworth-Heinemann, pp. 55–72.

Williamson PD, French JA, Thadani VM, Kim JH, Novelly RA, Spencer SS, Spencer DD and Mattson RH (1993) Characteristics of medial temporal lobe epilepsy: II. Interictal and ictal scalp electroencephalography, neuropsychological testing, neuroimaging, surgical results, and pathology. *Ann Neurol* **34**, 781–787.

Woo E, Chan YM, Yu YL, Chan YW and Huang CY (1988) If a well-stabilized epileptic patient has a subtherapeutic antiepileptic drug level, should the dose be increased? A randomized prospective study. *Epilepsia* **29**, 129–139.

Wyllie E, Luders H, Morris HH, Lesser RP and Dinner DS (1986) The lateralizing significance of versive head and eye movements during epileptic seizures. *Neurology* **36**, 606–611.

Wyllie E, Luders H, Morris HH III, *et al.* (1987) Clinical outcome after complete or partial cortical resection for intractable epilepsy *Neurology* **37**, 1634–1641.

Yaffe K and Lowenstein DH (1993) Prognostic factors of pentobarbital therapy for refractory generalized status epilepticus. *Neurology* **43**, 895–900.

Yahr MD, Sciarra D, Carter S and Merritt HH (1952) Evaluation of standard anticonvulsant therapy in three hundred nineteen patients. *J Am Med Assoc* **150**, 663–667.

Yerby MS (1992) Risks of pregnancy in women with epilepsy. *Epilepsia* **33** (Suppl 1), S23–S27.

Yerby MS, Van Belle G, Friel PN and Wilensky AJ (1987) Serum prolactins in the diagnosis of epilepsy: Sensitivity, specificity, and predictive value. *Neurology* **37**, 1224–1226.

Zuckerman EG and Glaser GH (1972) Urea-induced myoclonic seizures. *Arch Neurol* **27**, 14–28.

Zuk RF, Ginsberg VK, Houts T, Rabble J, Merrick H, Ullman EF, Fischer MM, Sizto CC, Stiso SN and Litman DJ (1985) Enzyme immunochromatography – a quantitative immunoassay requiring no instrumentation. *Clin Chem* **31**, 1144–1150.

Index

Page references in **bold** indicate key sections.